Misdirected Medicine

Misdirected Medicine

Dr. Sam McClatchie

WALKER AND COMPANY
New York

First published in the United States of America in 1973 by the Walker Publishing Company, Inc.

Published simultaneously in Canada by Fitzhenry & Whiteside, Limited, Toronto.

ISBN: 0-8027-0411-5

Library of Congress Catalog Card Number: 72-95770

Printed in the United States of America.

Contents

Preface

Dr. Samuel McClatchie

ANYONE WHO THINKS this book is an exposé of doctors will be disappointed. Most doctors I have met have been honest, well-motivated, competent and hard-working.

Sitting out here on the edge of the world, (this book was written while I had time on my hands in New Guinea), I flatter myself I have a different perspective on life. After forty years as a student and practitioner of medicine I have reluctantly concluded that much of what I have done has been a waste of time. The world is little better off and may soon be worse off than in my student days. I believe this is so because medicine—by which I mean the whole art and science of improving and preserving health, and not just that part of it performed by doctors of medicine—is on the wrong track.

We are heading for disaster if we keep on. That is my view. It is a view based on my own experiences in many parts of the world and on what I have heard and read from others. My book is not a deep scientific study. My references are newspapers, popular books on science and ecology and a very few standard medical publications. I have nothing else available out here. If some of my explanations—e.g., in atherosclerosis—seem vague and simplistic, I apologize to my colleagues. This is no place for a biochemical dissertation. The reader will find overlapping and repetition in various chapters. This is unavoidable since medicine does not come in compartments and life is an ecological whole.

I have no doubt that some people will agree with me entirely, some in part, and some will dismiss me as an old, outdated quack.

To these latter I say only that I qualified as a clinical pathologist in the United States, by examination of the American Board of Pathology, in October 1961. Thus I may be old but I can hardly be called either outdated or a quack.

The reader may wish to know where I have worked as a doctor. Though references to these countries will be noted in the book, I am including here a brief *curriculum vitae*, in which the first person singular, unavoidably, appears frequently.

I was born in Lurgan, Northern Ireland, on February 16, 1915. Among my first memories was the fighting between the I.R.A. and Protestant factions, which was as bad then as it is now.

In 1922 we emigrated to New Zealand, where I received primary school education.

In 1927 we moved to Toronto, Canada. I finished high school there and then entered the University of Toronto on a scholarship to study Biological and Medical Sciences, graduating B.A. in 1936 and M.D. in 1939.

In September 1939 I volunteered for war service with the Canadian Army and spent some time in Canada. I finally got overseas shortly after Pearl Harbor on a transfer to the Indian Medical Service. I served in the Middle East and Cyprus and then volunteered for Combined Operations with an Indian regiment. I landed in Sicily on D-Day and six weeks or so later hit the beach at Reggio Calabria twenty minutes after zero hour, which made me one of the first doctors to land in Europe. For the next two years I served in the 4th Indian Division as a Field Ambulance Company Commander, including the Battle of Cassino, and later with the 10th Indian Division in Northern Italy. I was awarded the Military Cross for a river crossing near Faenza late in 1944. Later I reached the rank of major.

I returned to Canada after V-E Day and spent three years in general practice in British Columbia. There I began specializing as a pathologist. As I wanted to do tropical medicine, I managed to get a commission in the U.S. Army, but with the onset of the Korean War I volunteered for combat duty and spent 1951 with the 25th Division in Korea.

PREFACE

I stayed with the U.S. Army for almost nine years. First I served in Korea, then in Japan as an advisor to the Japan Defense Force. Later I became a paratrooper and was Division Surgeon of the famous 82nd Airborne Division. Following an injury, I went back to pathology and general medicine for a while and then was sent to Taiwan as an advisor to the Chinese Nationalist Army.

From February 1957 to February 1959 I served in Formosa (Taiwan) and participated to some extent in the fight for the offshore islands of Quemoy and Matsu. I then returned to the U.S.A. and resigned from the Army to finish my training as a pathologist. My final rank was lieutenant colonel.

From 1959 to 1962 I trained in Vancouver, B.C., and then worked in New Zealand for a while as a pathologist.

In 1964 I went to Kenya and did tropical pathology for five years. Then, as my contract was over, I went to Sarawak for nine months, leaving because of illness in the family.

I took a post in Malawi for eighteen months and then went to New Guinea to participate in a new cancer-treatment unit as the pathologist. Due to staffing problems, the unit never really got going and I asked for my release. Recently I have been working in a hospital in Tanzania.

MISDIRECTED MEDICINE is thus based on my thirty-three years of experience as a doctor and has been rattling around in my head for a long time. The book is dogmatic and, I hope, provocative. I do not apologize for that. It has to be if I am to stir up enough interest to get medicine going in the right direction.

1

Bias and Blinkers — the Public Health Problem

1. Presidential Pressure

WHEN PRESIDENT FRANKLIN DELANO ROOSEVELT came to power in 1933 he was already partially paralyzed by poliomyelitis. The sight of the First Citizen of America in a wheel chair aroused tremendous sympathy, and he put his prestige behind the March of Dimes, which was a fund raised to treat the victims of the disease.

Epidemics of paralytic polio, especially when the respiratory muscles were paralyzed, really frightened people of the civilized world. I remember in the mid-1920s we had an epidemic in New Zealand in the summertime. Schools remained closed for two months after the usual holidays and, to my disgust, the local paper carried school lessons which my parents made me do. Every day I gargled with Condy's crystals (potassium permanganate) in solution and was fed Scott's Emulsion, only fractionally better than cod-liver oil. The worst part was the closing of all the movie theaters. Children were barred from all assemblies or social gatherings. Yet I enjoyed being out of school.

With the introduction of the Salk vaccine in 1955 and the live Sabin vaccine later, the incidence of paralytic disease dropped sharply. There were 13,850 paralytic cases in the United States in 1955. In 1969 there were 18. Today it no longer need be a menace. I say "need be" because, with fear gone, people neglect to have their children immunized. The Center for Disease Control of the United States government reported that in 1964 about 90 percent of American children between one and four years old had had polio vaccine. By 1969 it was down to 65 percent and in poverty areas was 50 percent. This is a clear case of neglect by both the public and the medical profession.

What has annoyed me most about the polio pressure over the last forty years is that while millions of dollars were being spent on it, other far more serious conditions were neglected. In 1936, at the height of Roosevelt's glory, the death rate in poliomyelitis epidemics ranged from 5 to 7 percent of the clinical cases. At the same time what was called summer diarrhea of infants was fatal in 30 to 40 percent of cases, due mainly to severe dehydration. Comparatively speaking, there should have been a March of Dollars for these poor kids, but they died and were buried quickly and the drums did not beat.

2. The Kind Killer

Probably the most consistent killer in human history is malaria. In 1955 it was estimated that there were 250 million cases with 2.5 million deaths annually. In 1956 the World Health Organization, with most nations cooperating, began a tremendous drive to kill the harmful mosquitoes, and in some areas the disease was wiped out. In others it could not be eliminated due to the logistical and ecological problems and the resistance of various human religious or tribal groups to spray programs. As might have been expected, insects became resistant to DDT and in South America and Vietnam some parasites developed resistance to commonly used drugs, though fortunately not entirely to quinine, the remedy first used by the ancient Incas.

In spite of these problems, it was estimated that by 1966, out of 1,576 million people previously exposed to malaria, 1,214 million lived in areas where the disease had been eradicated or the programs were in their last stages. Deaths had been reduced from 2.5 million to 1 million yearly. There still remained 300 million people in areas where little advance had been made due to factors mentioned above. I sometimes wonder if they and not the others are the fortunate ones.

In a symposium on malaria held at Walter Reed Army Medical Center in June 1966, Dr. L. J. Bruce-Chwatt, the Chief of the Research Division of Malaria Eradication of WHO, called malaria "the King Herod of the diseases of infants and children in undeveloped areas." He also said in another context, "We see the truth of the forecast that yesterday's triumphs will become tomorrow's headaches and realize that our task does not seem to have an end."

I believe that in 1972 this is already coming true. Since 1956 more than 10 million people are alive who would have died but for the efforts of the malariologists in prevention. Most of them were children when malaria was eliminated or reduced in their homeland. Now they are getting to the age where they too will have children. Some already have; and that is where the headache lies. Who will feed and clothe and educate this vast outpouring of human flesh onto the already impoverished lands where malaria once helped to keep the balance of nature? What sort of future do they face without jobs, without land to grow food, without hope for themselves and their children?

One of those areas is Bangla Desh, where 70 million people crowd into swampy deltas; where over 1 million were believed lost when a typhoon tidal wave broke the dikes and drowned them; where cholera killed hundreds of thousands and another 3 million were slaughtered in the Pakistan war before India stopped it;

where, as I write, a WHO official says there will be famine and bloodshed if we do not send money. What sort of life faces such people? I have seen them in Dacca and up-country. I have seen Calcutta, in Indian Bengal. I would not condemn any animal except a rat to live as those human beings do. I wonder if it would not be better, since the people cannot or will not control their fertility, if the malariologists would take their sprays and tablets and go home. It might be kinder in the end.

If the miracle should happen and we could get the world to adopt an ecologically balanced preventive health program with population control a major concern, then an all-out attack on malaria would be a wonderful thing. But what direction should it take? Elimination of the anopheles mosquito which carries malaria cannot be achieved by outdoor spraying because the sprays upset the balance of nature and kill useful animals. Indoor spraying helps but does not eradicate the carriers completely, especially when the insects become resistant. With a smaller world population we might treat all cases and give preventive drugs to others. However, malaria parasites are tenacious and they might survive in a few people to spread later or perhaps adapt themselves to other animals to reappear later in man. Some naturalists theorize that when Africans brought malaria across the Atlantic hundreds or even thousands of years ago, the parasites adapted themselves to New World monkeys and other animals. That shift could be reversed. Yellow fever still lurks in the high forests of Brazil, in the jungle monkeys and mosquitoes. Malaria could do the same.

Some say vaccines are the answer, provided people continue to take them and do not get lazy as they have done with polio and diphtheria, whooping-cough and tetanus immunizations. However, the malaria parasite is capable of antigenic variability, so that it might become resistant to a particular vaccine. Biological warfare to eliminate mosquitoes is another approach—perhaps the best one—but as yet nobody knows how. All things considered, it looks as if malaria is here to stay. Whenever military coups or small wars disrupt medical services the disease tends to break out again. The population explosion, combined with poverty and the indifference of leaders to the fate of the masses, makes it certain that epidemics will occur again. Nature has its own way of restoring the balance.

3. Deltas and Ditches

When John Foster Dulles reared up righteously and refused to give money and aid to President Nasser of Egypt for the construction of the Aswan Dam he was wiser, I am sure, than he ever suspected. The refusal was for political reasons. I am quite certain that if the Russians could have foreseen the consequences, they too would have refused.

It is easy to be what Americans call a "Monday-morning quarterback" telling his friends how the football team should have played on Saturday, but I think in this case, as in many similar projects, a good hard look at the long-term consequences might have prevented what may be a great disaster. The Egyptians have been worried that Israeli bombers might try to blow up the dam. If I were they, I'd be inclined to invite the Jews to do just that.

One major defect of dams, as beavers learned thousands of years ago, is that they silt up and form what in Canada we call a beaver meadow, a grassy plain where the lake used to be. This ends the dam's usefulness. It was probably the only problem considered in the preliminary planning of the new Aswan Dam (aside from flooding of archeological sites). What they did not foresee, or kept quiet about, was that, without the usual flushing out of delta lands, fresh silt would not be deposited, the delta would be less fertile, fertilizers would be required (to contaminate the water later) and, worse still, the salty seawater would seep back and ruin the fields.

Another consequence was the ruination of the shrimp fishing, since the shrimps also depended on this fresh material providing food for the tiny organisms on which they feed. Pollution from the great delta cities was worse; there was no great toilet flush each year to move the muck out into the Mediterranean.

All this was below the dam. The major disaster lies above it.

For 300 miles Lake Nasser extends south beyond Egypt into the Sudan. Two million acres of previously unusable land is now irrigable and is being brought into production in both countries. To do this requires farmers to settle, and these farmers are Egyptian and Sudanese peasants whose ideas of sanitation are primitive. The result is fouling of the waters and the introduction into the irrigation ditches of the eggs of bilharzia (schistosomiasis), which is the scourge of Egypt.

Statisticians say that this disease already costs Egypt £160 million a year in medical care and lost production. Every second Egyptian is infected. A conservative estimate is that the new dam could expose another 2 million people, of whom 70 percent could be infected. The snails that act as an intermediate host in the life cycle of the parasite infest the entire lake shore. It is only a matter of time before the disease spreads throughout this new homeland.

There is more. All this water-soaked area now provides an excellent breeding ground for Sudan's malaria-carrying mosquitoes and the sandfly that bites man and infects him with kala azar. As people travel to and from the area, they spread these diseases. Filarial parasites that cause elephantiasis can also grow well here. Hookworm has been found in 22.5 percent of people living in one of the newly developed areas, and the habit of defecating along the banks of a stream (for Muslim ablution purposes) will spread the disease among the barefoot fishermen who walk there.

Waste disposal in towns around the lake is another source of pollution. Medical experts are now calling for stringent public health measures. If they do not succeed—and I do not think they will in a nation as poorly disciplined as the Egyptians I knew—then the great Aswan High Dam may bring tragedy instead of prosperity to the people it serves.

The story is an old one. In China, along the Yangtze River, vast areas of rich alluvial soil were unusable because of schistosomiasis and malaria. The Communists claim to have eradicated the snails that carry the former and the mosquitoes that cause the latter. Perhaps they have, but no Westerner, to my knowledge, has reported on the problem since they came to power. Certainly it would have required tremendous discipline and a great public health program. If they achieved it, then they, at least in this regard, are heading in the right direction. Somebody needs to. There are already 50 million people in the world who have one or more of the three main forms of bilharzia.

4. The Freeloaders

The schistosomes, filariases and some other types of worm spend the human part of their cycle within the body tissues. However, there are others that stay most of their lives in the intestine and these I call the freeloaders. Nobody knows how many people carry these unwanted passengers and very little is being done about them. The ascaris or roundworm is everywhere. The incidence in the Orient is thought to be about 90 percent. In the southeastern United States over 30 percent of people in certain areas are infested. This worm does not often cause overt disease unless so numerous as to block the intestine. It does interfere with absorption of dietary protein—i.e., it steals food a child sorely needs.

The real killer among these worms is hookworm. In 1947 Dr. N. R. Stoll estimated that 456 million people had them. We could probably double that figure today with the increase in population. There are two kinds, but their effects are similar. They are found in all the warmer, wetter parts of the world from Africa and Asia to the southern United States. Both hookworm and roundworm are spread by bad sanitary habits and, in some countries, by using "night soil" to fertilize vegetable gardens.

Along with malaria, which breaks down the red blood cells, the hookworm, which hooks onto the intestinal wall and sucks blood, is responsible for much of the severe anemia seen in the tropics. In North America normal human beings have about 15 grams of hemoglobin to each 100 milliliters of blood. When the proportion drops under 12 grams we begin to wonder and at 10 grams the patient is definitely anemic. Anyone known to be down to 6 grams would be rushed to a hospital on a stretcher, yet in New Guinea every day pregnant women, further depleted by the demands of their babies, walk into a hospital with less than that. In fact, at least once a week we have someone with a hemoglobin count of 1.5 to 2 grams—i.e., 10 to 15 percent of normal. I saw the same thing in Africa and Asia.

Unfortunately, we doctors cannot do much about this disease. We have drugs to eliminate both roundworm and hookworm from the intestines, but the barefoot patient goes home to walk on contaminated ground and get hookworm again, or uses unsanitary habits and gets roundworm eggs into his mouth once more. Some immunity to hookworm is believed to develop after the first infection, but anemic and malnourished people do not develop it as well as the healthy person. If reinfection can be avoided, 70 percent of the hookworms die off in a year or so and they are all gone in five to fifteen years.

If we could put shoes on all the people where hookworm is found, the disease would disappear, since the larvae, hatching out of the eggs, penetrate the skin that touches the contaminated ground. The disease has lessened greatly in the southern United States because most poor people today do wear shoes. The current fad for going barefoot is stupid when living in hot countries such as New Guinea, yet young and old Australians are doing it every day.

Elimination of roundworms is more difficult. It would require a world-wide education program, a complete overhaul of sanitary customs and facilities and then mass treatment to get rid of the worms we already have. As far as I know, such a massive program has not been tried. If it were, it would also eliminate schistosomiasis. The results in better health, more productivity and reduction of medical expenses would be fantastic, provided population control was started at the same time.

5. The Proximity Fuse

To the average American, tuberculosis is something his grandfather may have died of, his father probably was exposed to, but he does not need to worry about. In the undeveloped countries the people are still back in his grandfather's day. There are about 20 million infectious cases in the world today and in some areas the morbidity is estimated at 1 percent.

Tuberculosis is usually transmitted by droplets coughed or spat out by those who are infected. That is why I call it the proximity fuse. It explodes on close contact. Consequently, people living under poor conditions, crowded into small, badly ventilated huts, are likely to get it and spread it. The situation is made worse nowadays with the drift of poor people to the cities. The disease is rife in the favelas (slums) of Rio and São Paulo, Brazil; in the shanty towns of Africa; in the squatter settlements around major towns of Asia and New Guinea. It is further aggravated because many of the country people coming to live in these slums have never been exposed to the disease—e.g., the Highlanders of New Guinea coming to coast towns—and they have no resistance.

In most countries there are surveys and TB treatment programs. The problem is that curing the disease takes a long time. Injections and pills must be taken regularly for months and resistance to drugs may develop. Following up such cases and persuading them to come back for review is a job demanding unending patience. The victims often feel well and quit treatment before they are cured, only to relapse months or years later. Let me give some examples.

It is reported that in Paris, France, 25 percent of newly discovered cases of TB vanish from the clinics in the first year of treatment. In Japan 40 percent of cases have become resistant to treatment because of poor supervision, absenteeism and so on. In primitive New Guinea, where the rate of TB in coastal areas is 1 percent, the situation is better. Because the Highlanders were isolated and free of TB until they began coming to the coastal plantations to work, a strong TB-prevention program was set up. By law, any known case had to take two years of treatment with injections of streptomycin and oral drugs three times weekly. Anyone who defected and ran off to his village was brought back by the police. What will happen when independence comes I do not know, but it is likely to be as in Africa, where discipline is almost non-existent.

The Communist countries such as Hungary have laws that enforce treatment. They have less of a problem. The Chinese, who used to be plagued with the disease, now claim to have almost eliminated it. With discipline that is quite possible. In the more relaxed countries of the West and in the poor non-Communist countries the disease is likely to increase as the drift to the cities continues.

6. The Bug Bites Back

When I went on the wards in 1936 pneumonia was a dreaded disease. We used to grow pneumococci from the sputum, determine what type they were and then inject the patient with the specific antiserum. It worked if the patient could live long enough to get the serum. We had prevention for diphtheria but no drugs if somebody got the disease. It took about a year of painful heavy-metal injections to cure syphilis. No drug would cure TB. Prontosil, an early sulfonamide, was just becoming available for treatment of previously deadly streptococcal infections such as puerperal fever. Then in 1938 sulfapyridine was discovered and pneumococcal pneumonia was no longer so deadly.

Since the Second World War the Age of Antibiotics has arrived. In the developed countries infectious diseases are now far down the list of causes of death. But they may not stay there. In other chapters I mention the dangers of ill-advised use of antibiotics which has resulted in many people becoming sensitized to the drugs and unable to take them again. Another major danger is the resistance which some bacteria acquire to an antibiotic that previously prevented their proliferation or actually killed them. It has recently been shown that bacteria can transfer resistance directly from one to another, even of different tribes—for example, from the non-pathogenic E. coli to the pathogenic Salmonella (such as typhoid). This is a very disturbing discovery which makes it imperative that we control the use of antibiotics far more strictly than we do now.

A third problem is only now coming to light: the toxic effects of the chemicals after prolonged use. We will see more of this as the years pass.

According to Drs. Lawrence Garrod and Francis O'Grady in their excellent book *Antibiotic and Chemotherapy*, "it seems unlikely that any totally new antibiotic remains to be discovered, since those of recent origin have similar properties to others already known. It therefore will be wise to husband our resources, and employ them in such a way as to preserve them." In other words, we will be in a mess if because of our misuse of these drugs, bacteria become resistant to them all. Garrod and O'Grady go on to say, "The community has to be considered, since it has been abundantly proved that the more some antibiotics are used, the less useful do they become, because the frequency of bacterial resistance to them increases correspondingly."

To prevent this they advise certain procedures: certain drugs must be restricted to use only when no other antibiotic will work; when resistance appears, switch to another effective antibiotic; prescribe a wide variety of drugs, all for short times only, so resistance does not develop; use combinations known, in certain cases, not to cause resistance. This sort of policy requires interference by a Public Health Department into the sacred field of treatment by individual doctors and can rouse the ire of the drug companies. It has been pursued by some regional authorities. We shall see if our leaders have the courage to make it national and international policy.

7. Will the Hockey Stick Come Back?

Sex is here to stay and since it is we had better take a good look at the VD situation. When I was a young medical student I worked one summer in a lumber camp. The men were rough, tough and uneducated. Once a month they got to town for a few days and blew their pay on liquor and women. As one said to me, "Look, son, you ain't a man till you've had a coupla doses." That attitude seems to be coming back.

In those days there were no sulfa drugs and no antibiotics. Treatment of syphilis took at least a year of mercurial and arsenical drugs by weekly injections. Treatment of gonorrhea by instillation of various silver solutions and argyrol (silver proteinate) was considered a great advance. Potassium-permanganate flushing of the passages was another procedure, and when the inevitable strictures ensued in chronic cases, we young medics were instructed in the gentle art of pushing an ever larger series of long, curved probes up the urethra into the bladder of the squirming subject. We called these torture instruments "hockey sticks" and we wondered why on earth anyone would risk getting VD if he knew the consequences. However, the urge is primeval and the parade went on. It could start all over again.

There are only a few places left in the world—such as the Highlands of New Guinea, which were not reached by the white man until the late 1920s—where syphilis is uncommon. Unfortunately, "progress" will not be denied and so one more advantage of civilization is reaching a primitive people. Gonorrhea goes with it.

After World War II, when penicillin became available to all, it was thought that venereal disease would be eliminated and join smallpox in the history books. Today it has sprung back to epidemic proportions. In 1970 in the United States gonorrhea took second place to the common cold as the most common communicable disease. And that, please remember, was on the basis of only the reported cases. In 1971, out of a population of about 20 million, half a million Canadians were said to be suffering from VD. Many of them did not know it or ignored it. Most of the cases were gonorrhea, but syphilis was increasing too.

The U.S. Public Health Service, commenting on a survey of private physicians in 1968, claimed that these doctors reported only between 12 and 19 percent of the infectious syphilis cases they treated and between 11 and 17 percent of the gonorrhea cases, even though all states have laws requiring reporting of VD. Like an ice cube in a highball, most of the problem was below the surface. It was estimated that in 1972 there would be 624,000 new cases of VD reported in the United States. The actual figure was expected to be over 2 million.

The situation in Europe is variable. In 1971 among the porno-permissive Danes there were 319 reported cases of VD per 100,000 people. The casual Swedes had a rate of 514 per 100,000 and beat the Californians to the top of the dungheap. The greatest percentages of cases were in men aged 20-24 years and girls of 18-19, the ages when the sex drive is strongest and optimism highest.

In Russia in 1971 the Supreme Soviet made refusal to accept treatment a crime and increased the jail sentences for transmission of VD. The Chinese Communists claim to have eliminated it and several eminent Western doctors, including Dr. Paul Dudley White of Boston, agree that their claim is true in all but a few areas of the country. From this it would seem that as Western customs became more liberal and the Chinese more puritanical, the incidence of VD rose in the West and dropped in the East. However, Dr. William F. Schwartz, Chief of the Educational Services Unit of the Venereal Diseases Branch of the Center for Disease Control of the U.S.A., stated in 1971 that "there's no evidence to indicate sexual behavior is any different today than it was fifteen years ago." There is a freer discussion of sex and more permissiveness in books and movies but not necessarily more intercourse.

The Pill probably made people feel freer to have sex. A survey in Sweden showed that 36 percent of women with gonorrhea had had more frequent sexual intercourse and with four times as many partners after they went on the Pill. One effect is undisputed: the use of condoms has decreased. Sex, like "skinny dipping" in a river, is more spontaneous and more fun when done *au naturel*. Unfortunately, it makes transmission of disease much easier. The condom did present a barrier to bacteria.

Another problem is recognition of disease. Most men who get VD are aware of it, but it is claimed that 80 percent of women who have gonorrhea do not have enough symptoms to seek medical attention. It may be wishful thinking, but they tend to look upon a vaginal discharge as just another woman's problem, a natural cross to bear.

All this is bad enough. We are now running into the difficulties I mentioned earlier in Section 6 above. Gonococci are becoming increasingly resistant to antibiotics. Today in some countries it takes three or four times the dose of penicillin that it took in 1958 to cure gonorrhea. Other antibiotics that were effective are now of little use. The bug became resistant to sulfa drugs years ago, but fortunately that resistance has decreased somewhat due to lack of use. The rules I mentioned in Section 6 will have to be enforced if we are to be successful with treatment. There is an additional rule: treatment sufficient to cure gonorrhea may suppress syphilis so that the patient does not know he has it. A blood test to rule it out is mandatory six months after treatment for gonorrhea.

Experts are working on various aspects of the problem. A serologic test to detect gonorrhea would be of great help, especially in females. Vaccines for prevention of the several venereal diseases are also a hope for the future. In the meantime it looks as if discipline is the answer, as it is in China: discipline in sexual customs and methods; discipline in case reporting and contact investigation; discipline in treatment, with elimination of bootlegged antibiotics and half-hearted measures. Until then VD rates will go in only one direction: up.

8. Affluent Effluence

The title of this section is a play on words. By one definition it means "flowing freely, flowing out." By another, "wealthy, flowing out." I mean all of this. It is primarily the outflow from our wealthy society, flowing without hindrance, that is our greatest single problem today, a problem that now overshadows our previous fears of annihilation by the hydrogen bomb.

So much has been written about this that I am not going to

discuss it except in relation to our medical problems. Lake Erie is already almost a cesspool. As I write this, Jacques Cousteau says the Mediterranean Sea is dying, with animal and plant life reduced to a fraction of what it was thirty years ago. Thor Heyerdahl reported mid-ocean pollution so bad he couldn't brush his teeth with mid-Atlantic seawater on his *Ra II* voyage. We have all read about the oil slicks polluting beaches. DDT has been found in Antarctic penguins and mercury in swordfishes in the Atlantic and South Pacific. On land we have air pollution. In September 1971 I was in the United States with my family. We flew from Washington, D.C., to New York on a sunny Sunday morn and I couldn't see the ground for smog. Down below, if I had fallen into the water made famous by the calendar picture "September Morn," I'd have needed an antityphoid shot and gamma globulin to be sure I didn't get hepatitis. This is what we have done to our earth, the only home we will ever have.

We are already reaping the results of our folly. Emphysema and cancer of the lung are disabling or killing millions of people each year. This is partly due to smoking, but air pollution is a partner in the crime. Air pollution is a public health problem, whereas smoking is, in some degree, a personal problem. It involves big business far more than smoking does and so it will be harder to regulate because of the expense involved. Once regulated, it may be easier to control than smoking, which is an addiction, not subject to logic.

Water and land pollution have two main aspects. The first is control of human and animal wastes. These are not intrinsically harmful. They overwhelm the natural processes of biodegradation by sheer volume. It will cost more, but we already know how to take care of these wastes, returning valuable organic matter to the soil whence it came. The second aspect is the control of man-made products. I do not refer to such things as bottles, boxes, car bodies and so on. I am worried about the new chemicals that pour onto our land and end in our streams. Some are obviously harmful, as, for example, the chemicals that killed millions of fish in the Rhine in 1971 and the detergents that frothed out of septic tanks or piled up in bubbly drifts on rivers of the United States some years back. Others have no known harmful effects . . . not yet. But what will happen twenty or more years from now? It is not inconceivable that we are already absorbing substances in our water supply that will kill us all.

In the recent furor in Australia over imipramine, which was suspected of deforming babies as thalidomide did (and reported by the same obstetrician), the head of the Drug Evaluation Committee of the Australian government said so many drugs were reaching the market that there were insufficient inspectors to examine them closely. Consequently, the committee had to read reports from elsewhere and study the manufacturers' specifications and tests and decide on that basis whether or not to license distribution. Now, if we have that much trouble with drugs designed specifically for human consumption, how can we possibly monitor the hundreds of thousands of chemicals that are the waste products of industrial processes and that are gotten rid of in the least expensive way, which usually means dumping in the nearest river? Some companies put such products down deep wells. But who can be sure there is no leakage now or will be none after a minor earth movement?

The truth of the matter is that in our materialistic greed we are taking chances with our health, our lives and our world. Nobody working in the medical professions should forget this for a minute and, while we cannot change laws overnight, we owe it to our consciences to make sure everyone else knows we do not approve of what is going on.

Government agencies are swamped with other work. There is some research on these pollution problems by universities and private agencies, such as research laboratories of commercial companies interested in particular products. Broadly speaking, the field has been neglected until now and the sheer complexity of it would daunt even the keenest medical biochemist with a dozen computer experts to help him. Nevertheless, the problems must be tackled. Medical scientists cannot afford to neglect them any longer. At the moment we have two alternatives. One is to declare a moratorium on production of all new chemicals right now, and that will not be done as long as our society has "growthandprogress" as its goal. The other is to insist that no waste product of any industry be put where it can contaminate the environment. The breaking down of such wastes to basic harmless elements will be very expensive. What other alternative do we have?

9. Who Gets the Gravy?

Even in America there is only so much real money. There are so many scientists, so many technicians to go around. Problems must be allocated priorities, which leads to the question: Who gets the gravy?

I have already shown in Section 1 above what can happen when special pleaders get their way. It is still going on. We have nationwide programs for sufferers from phenylketonuria (PKU)—which occurs in about one in 7,000 births—for cystic fibrosis, disseminated sclerosis and many other unusual diseases, programs usually started by someone whose relative has been afflicted. This is all very well, but the time has come to look at the overall picture and allocate proper priorities. The U.S. Army Medical Corps has a motto, "The Greatest Good to the Greatest Number." Whether we like it or not, we are in a war for survival, and, in my opinion, that motto should be everybody's motto. We literally do not have the time or facilities to waste on relatively unimportant diseases.

Prestige projects are not confined to building dams or bridges or convention halls in developing countries. There are prestige projects in medicine too. New Guinea offers a prime example. Several years ago it was decided that treatment for cancer patients should be modernized. With the advice of Australian and international experts, a radiotherapy center which uses the cobalt bomb was designed and built in Lae. The unit itself cost roughly A$200,000 and the running costs are A$57,000 per year. I was recruited to do the pathology for the center and for the hospitals in New Guinea Territory (not Papua). When I arrived my technician had left. No other could be recruited. The radiotherapist and maxillofacial surgeon both went off to greener fields and the gynecologist was transferred. Replacements were not available. The unit sat there with a surgeon trying to run it as well as a heavy surgical service while a radiotherapist came up from Australia every few months, a quite unsatisfactory situation. Even when it was in operation the unit treated only about 140 patients per year because the cost of transporting patients by air from elsewhere in the territory (often the only way) was prohibitive.

The cost of treating one patient in this institution was A$407, which is an unacceptably high figure in a poor country. Sentimentalists may cry, "How can you put a value on a human life?" but in fact we can and do, as any old soldier will certify. Even in peacetime, governments allocate a limited amount for equipping and staffing hospitals and the very fact of doing so puts a value on lives: lives lost because there is no equipment for heart surgery, lives lost because kidney transplants cannot be done, and so on. The bad thing about the New Guinea project was that spending the same amount of money on a TB program or on child health would have saved many more, and younger, lives than the cobalt bomb ever could.

Recently there was another report on health care in undeveloped countries. In September 1972 Dr. James McGilivray, Director of the Christian Medical Commission of the World Council of Churches, was quoted by the *Medical Tribune* as saying, regarding money paid out for maintenance of medical missions, "As much as 90 percent of this is misplaced." As the churches invest about £5-7 million annually in medical missions and the annual operating costs are over £120 million, these are colossal sums to waste.

According to this report, medical missions provide 30 to 40 percent of medical care in the developing world, and the need for a change of direction is urgent. Biomedical technology which requires expensive hospitals and equipment for its implementation can have only a limited impact on the total health need. Dr. McGilivray said, "But the fact that we have limited effectiveness in this area does not seem to deter us from continuing with this enormous and at times unavailing effort—building even more and even larger institutions."

Dr. McGilivray produced data to show that a health center could be built for £20,000, the cost of only four beds in a teaching hospital, and it would provide most of the health-care requirements for 20,000 people. About 250 such health centers, enough for the entire population of Zambia, could be built for what it cost to build a newly completed teaching hospital in Lusaka, the capital of Zambia.

To give an idea of health-care delivery costs per illness treated: The cost in a dispensary (health sub-center) per illness is 9 pence; in a primary health center, 22 pence; in a district hospital, £4.72; in a central hospital, £20.80. Admittedly, more serious cases can be handled in the central hospital, serious in the sense of cancers, degenerative diseases, orthopedic problems and so on. However, while we experts busy ourselves with these human wrecks, how many others die of curable conditions out in the bush because there is no medical assistant in a health center nearby?

Modern medicine is the direct descendant of ancient Western medicine in which emphasis was primarily on cures rather than prevention. It still is. This, I submit, is really misdirected. Surgery to me is an admission of failure: failure to cure cancer by drugs; or, better still, to prevent it; failure to curb the slaughter on the highways by medically designed safety measures; failure to eliminate the causes of arteriosclerosis so that aortic transplants and vessel grafts would be unnecessary. Medical treatment too is often failure: failure to insist on inoculations against infectious disease; failure to eliminate parasites such as bilharzia from water; failure most of all in bringing home to our people what they do to themselves by improper living habits. But all these diseases get priority for treatment, either surgical or medical. The surgeons and physicians, the hospitals and outpatient clinics all get the funds, and, in proportion, preventive services are ignored and impoverished. Yet with proper preventive medicine we could close up half the hospitals we now fill with patients as we closed the

TB sanitaria after the Second World War. The title of this chapter is "Bias and Blinkers." We are biased in the way we handle medical problems and we cannot see the whole view but only the narrow roadway we have always trod.

In an article entitled "Where Doctors Fail," published in the *Saturday Review* of August 22, 1970, Dr. John H. Knowles, General Director of the Massachusetts General Hospital and Professor of Medicine at Harvard Medical School, said, "The system must be changed from the present last-line-of-defense, acute care, essentially passive approach to one that stresses preventive and rehabilitative services." Later he said, "At the same time, medicine should be at the forefront on larger issues affecting public health, such as population and pollution control." This is from the director of one of the most famous curative institutions in the world. He is getting the gravy, but he knows where it should really be going. Diogenes would have loved him.

2

The Nut Lab

1. Foibles and Fallacies

IN THE U.S. ARMY DURING THE MID-1950's there was a Nutrition Laboratory at Fitzsimons Army Hospital. Those who did not work in it called it the Nut Lab. Looking back, I am inclined to think the name was uncomfortably close to the truth.

While I was there, reports began coming from American advisors in Taiwan that many Chinese Nationalist Army soldiers were night blind, supposedly due to years of privation during the campaigns on the mainland. This was years before President Nixon started cuddling up to Mao Tse-tung and we of the Medical Corps were concerned about the fitness of the Nationalist soldiers. Generalissimo Chiang Kai-shek kept talking about returning to the mainland, and those of us who had been held back from chasing the running Reds in June 1951 were convinced that we should finish them off before they regained their strength and overran Southeast Asia. They did overrun Tibet and bloodied India's nose before turning the task over to the North Vietnamese.

The Nut Lab was asked to send a team of experts out to Taiwan. They went and did a lot of biochemical checking on diets and serum tests on the soldiers. They concluded that the stories were untrue except for a very few cases and recommended that the traditional white rice be supplemented by a multivitamin liquid to make sure. The result was a yellowish cast to the rice, and the soldiers raised hell about it. They would not eat brown, unpolished rice, that was for animals, and they did not want the "long noses' " new yellow additive. The rumor spread that it would destroy their manhood. I was by that time in Taiwan and got caught up in the controversy since I was an advisor to the Chinese Army Medical Corps.

The whole investigation, with a repeat done several years later, cost a lot of money and was quite unnecessary. The Army eye specialist at Fitzsimons was not consulted. He told me he could have seen retinal changes indicative of deficiency by a simple eye examination. Old soldiers on Taiwan laughed about the whole business. We knew the men did not like going on night maneuvers due to fear of spirits or to simple laziness. As I said to a friend, "They can go through the deepest night and find their way to the grog shop or the cat house with no trouble. Whoever believes they are night blind is gullible."

Centuries ago the Chinese made white rice a status symbol and fed the husks to the pigs. The pigs were healthy as a result. What saved the Chinese was that they ate the pigs and so got the good of the rice secondhand . . . if they could afford to buy pork. If they were too poor and ate white rice and little else, they were likely to get beriberi.

Similarly, for people living on a maize diet there is the possibility of a deficiency of nicotinic acid, one of the B-complex vitamins. The result is pellagra, a disease well known in the southern United States in the old days. It is seen in Africa today, where maize is the staple cereal, so much so that most Bantu claim it is "their" food and do not know that it came originally from America. To make matters worse, they insist that white maize is the only sort fit to eat, thus losing the Vitamin A content of the yellow variety. I saw this in Kenya during a maize crop failure when the Africans protested that the yellow maize sent from the United States as famine relief gave them a bellyache and was not nutritious.

Those who followed the war of the Nigerian government against the Ibos read much about the malnutrition that resulted and the deaths of thousands of children from kwashiorkor. Even in peacetime kwashiorkor is one of the greatest killers of children in Africa. It is also seen under other names in India, Central America and Southeast Asia.

In Malawi and New Guinea such malnutrition of children is common, especially in those weaned some months previously. I had assumed it was due to poverty, but the pediatricians assured me the mothers were healthy and there was no real food shortage. Local customs prescribe giving these infants mushy concoctions of starches which fill their stomachs and ease their hunger but do not supply enough protein of adequate quality. Most primitive peoples are not aware that foods contain different nutrients and that children need a variety for growth and development. If these pot-bellied little fellows live long enough to eat what adults eat, they recover unless, as happens in wartime or famine, there is a genuine food shortage. If there are too many kids in the family, of course their chances are reduced.

This was brought out in 1971 in a study by Dr. Adolfo Chavez, head of the Nutrition Division of Mexico's National Institute of Nutrition. He found that poverty was not the sole governing factor in nutrition. Ignorance of modern concepts of health was important. Malnourished children were more often seen in large families where babies were often weaned early because the mother was pregnant again. The new babies were all right at first, but eventually the mother's milk was insufficient and they fell behind other children. Feeding supplements to a similar group of pregnant women and later to the babies resulted in higher birth weights, greater consumption of mother's milk and more normal development.

Kwashiorkor is basically due to a lack of proper proteins. When the child is weaned he is deprived of the proteins and immune bodies of his mother's milk. His own immunity to disease is not well developed and so, crawling about, he may pick up gastroenteritis, measles, hookworm, schistosomiasis and other diseases.

Diarrhea is common as the result of infection and prevents absorption of what protein he does get or what his normal intestinal flora might provide. The result is a listless, puffy, weak child with a fatty liver, who will either succumb to infection or peter out like an engine out of gas.

Public health authorities in the United States profess great concern about poor nutrition. They do not do as much as they should about it. For example, we all know that whole-wheat bread is better than white. But does anyone ban white bread? No. The manufacturers add synthetic vitamin mixtures and softeners, slice it and package it, then charge more while trumpeting their virtues to the skies. They should be sued by the Department of Health for putting out an inferior food and by the Department of Culture, if we ever have one, for an insult to the arts of cooking and gastronomy.

2. Up with Cholesterol

Most of us seem to be gullible where nutrition is concerned. When I was a medical student I was told that human beings needed good-quality animal proteins and fats because we could not manufacture certain amino acids and fatty acids we required and vegetables were deficient in them. The virtue of plenty of milk and butter and steaks was unquestioned. I wonder how many millions of people have died because of that. Even the experience of the European countries in the Second World War did not shake our faith in the Great American Diet. There, when put on drastically reduced amounts of milk, butter, eggs, meat and refined sugars and limited to a basic ration, it was found that fewer people were having heart attacks and strokes and their general health was better than before the war. When the war ended, the Europeans went back to their "better diet" and the heart attacks and strokes rose even higher than their pre-war levels.

It has been said that high cholesterol levels in our blood, due to our diet, are the cause of the heart attacks. The plaques that form in the arteries are made up of cholesterol-rich fatty compounds. However, the biochemical linkages are far too complicated to be discussed in this book and there is a lot of argument as to just what happens. All I want to say about it here is that, quite inadvertently, man may have interfered with nature and brought us to our present condition by something he did thousands of years ago.

Early man was a hunter and gatherer. He ate the meat of animals of the forest and parkland. Then he tamed cattle and moved out into the grasslands which had been cleared by fires set by himself or caused by lightning. That was when the trouble began.

Herbivorous animals live on grass or leaves. Some take both if available. About 1968, in a study reported in the *British Medical Journal*, Dr. Crawford of the Nuffield Foundation analyzed the meat of domestic cattle, wild game in East Africa, zoo animals and man. The results were astonishing. I talked to him about it when he came to Malawi for a visit in 1970.

There are two main kinds of vegetation—oil-rich leaves, which are high in unsaturated fats, and water-rich grass, which is poorly supplied with such fats. When the lean meat (containing fats and proteins) of giraffes and buffaloes that lived in forest land and ate a lot of leaves was compared with the meat of those living on grassland or fed grass in zoos, he found tremendous differences in the amount and types of fat in their muscles. Like domestic cattle, the grass-fed animals were low in unsaturated fats and high in saturated ones. Civilized man's muscle was essentially similar to the domestic cattle he ate.

Today we eat meat of animals fed almost entirely on grass. So we are deprived of a good supply of vitally necessary unsaturated fats. Our diet, in that sense, is unnatural as compared with that of the ancient hunter. In an article I wrote in 1969 which did not find a publisher, I recommended that the Chicago stockyards should provide a leafy diet to the steers in their feeding pens so that the lazy human consumer would get his quota of unsaturated fats in his steak. The taste might be a bit different, but we spray hickory-flavored aerosols on our barbecues, so why not have the steak pre-flavored and more nutritious?*

"All right," you agree, "let's have the unsaturated fats. Why do we need them anyway?"

"Because if we don't get enough of them and get too many saturated fats, we are likely to get arteriosclerosis," I reply. "Saturated fats and cholesterol seem to go together in this disease."

There is good evidence that our diet is at least one of the reasons we get arteriosclerosis. Most animals do not live long enough to show the effects, which is why we think they do not have the disease. Until fairly recently neither did man. Elephants living in the Tsavo, in Kenya, where they have killed most of the trees and have to live on grass, are now showing similar plaques in their arteries as they get old enough.

There are other theories as to the reason for arteriosclerosis. One is that stress of modern living has its effect. Another is that eating refined sugars and carbohydrates is the cause. There is a complex linkage of fat and carbohydrate metabolism in our bodies that is not completely understood, so perhaps refined carbohydrates are also gumming up the works. At any rate, something is drastically wrong with our civilized diet, in more ways than one, as I discuss in Chapter 12. I would add only one more story here.

In the Highlands of New Guinea the uncivilized Melanesians live on a diet of kau-kau (sweet potatoes) and leafy vegetables. Wild animals have been hunted almost to extinction, so their meat is a rare delicacy. Pigs are kept, but are killed *en masse* at rare intervals for ceremonial banquets. Preliminary studies on the nutrition of these peoples show that on their ordinary diet they are in negative nitrogen balance: in other words, they are losing more

* Today Australian government research workers are feeding cattle unsaturated oil supplements to see if the unsaturated fat content of the meat can be raised and still remain palatable by modern standards.

nitrogen, which is the basis of proteins, in bodily excretions than they take in with their low-protein diet. How can this be? How can they be healthy, especially as they cannot be getting the necessary proteins in their food?

One theory is that, like the nitrogen-fixing bacteria that form nodules in the roots of clover, supplying the plant with nitrogen, there are nitrogen-fixing bacteria in the intestines of these people. Perhaps the bacteria derive their nitrogen from atmospheric nitrogen dissolved in the person's blood. They then manufacture amino acids for their own use with this nitrogen, and when they die, the bacteria are digested by their host, who absorbs thereby the required building blocks for his proteins. It appears that this is a symbiotic relationship made possible by the vegetarian diet. At any rate, here are healthy people, with no arteriosclerosis, living on what our experts say is an inadequate diet. So much for experts!

3. In the Midst of Plenty

New Zealand is one of the richest countries in the world, agriculturally—a land of milk and honey. Yet when I went back as a pathologist to the area I had lived in as a boy, I was surprised to find that nutritional anemia was fairly common among young Maori children, who were numerous in that district. It was not due to poverty—New Zealand is a welfare state. It was due to ignorance of what to feed babies after they left the breast. The result was folic acid and Vitamin C deficiency, which produced severe anemia.

This was another example of bad dietary practices such as I saw in Malawi and New Guinea. Here it was in the context of a European-style diet, but a badly chosen one. Fish and chips, washed down with sweet carbonated beverages, is a common meal and there is money for white bread, sweet biscuits and so on for the toothless infant to mumble on. In New Guinea, on the coast, I have seen mothers feeding tiny infants on such biscuits and "lolly water," as the Australians call soft drinks. Too much of that sort of diet could be fatal.

America does not escape. Similar ignorance of reasonable diet principles is common. It is not solely lack of money or education. In a recent study, dentists were concerned about the rising incidence of periodontal disease in American children. The cause is not known, but I am willing to bet it has something to do with the consumption of candies, soft drinks and ice-cream confections plus a lack of good hearty chewing material in the daily diet. It is long past time for us to take a critical look at our food habits.

4. Malthus and Malnutrition

Dogmatically speaking, malnutrition is a self-inflicted disease in most cases. Therefore the sufferer deserves little sympathy. I can hear howls of protest: "What about the kids? It isn't their fault." It isn't, but when the same kids grow up and do exactly what their parents did, it is time to ponder whether or not we should have felt sorry for them ten years previously. Periodically we are told by WHO and other world bodies that two thirds of the human race go hungry to bed each night. Whose fault is that? Who has all these kids? Somebody called government? Or *them*? Every adult knows where kids come from and what causes them. He knows too how to prevent it, in one way or another. We make much of the "freedom of the individual" and his right to decide his own life. Why then do we feel it necessary to bail him out when he gets into trouble through exercising that freedom?

A short time ago an agronomist was awarded a Nobel Prize for producing a miracle wheat that would give several times the yield of previous varieties. He was widely hailed as a savior of starving millions in India and elsewhere. The Green Revolution was at hand and the Hindu farmers could eat a square meal again. I felt about him the way I feel about the discoverer of DDT until I read an interview in which he said, in effect, that his discovery might buy time until the world came to its senses and controlled its population. That statement alone made the award worthwhile. Here was a man who understood the real cause of most malnutrition.

There is a wry comment on malnutrition and expert opinions which I discovered after writing this book. For years we have been sending milk powder and other concentrated milk products to famine areas as a major weapon in our battle against hunger. For years the ungrateful recipients have complained that these products were not good food and gave them bloating and abdominal discomfort. Our experts put this down to cultural prejudice.

Now, it appears, many peoples of the world such as Chinese, other Asians and some Africans, who do not drink milk after leaving their mother's breast, have been shown to lack the enzyme that breaks down lactose, the milk sugar, into simpler sugars. The enzyme seems to disappear after weaning. For such people milk is relatively indigestible and their complaints are justified. We Europeans have retained the enzyme, probably as a result of social and genetic selection. Our nutritionists apparently never considered that other people could be different—or dare I say that they didn't want to consider it in our "equality-obsessed" United Nations?

5. Supplements, Sprays and Safety

Mass production is the way of life in the Western world. It started with cars and ended with carcasses—not human, although we get them too on the highways.

Feed-lot fattening of steers by conveyor-belt systems; battery raising of chickens, crammed four to a twelve-by-eighteen-inch cage; automatic planting, spraying and processing of millions of lettuce heads in great fields—all are manifestations of our genius for production which enables us to grow more food with fewer employees than any other country in the world. It may be old age—I remember my father complaining years ago—but somehow steaks don't taste as good, chickens are too bland and lettuce is blah nowadays. I could put up with that, but now whenever I bite an apple I wonder what I am eating on the skin. When I slice a capon I wonder if the hormones are all absorbed and gone. When I eat the blotting paper "untouched by human hands" that is called bread I wonder what the added "freshener" will do to me.

In July 1971 Ralph Nader's group put out another of his famous reports, this one on agricultural products. He stated that annually one billion pounds of pesticides are sprayed on farm crops in the United States. Some of this ends in our bodies, either directly from the vegetables or concentrated through the animals we eat which ate the plants. In addition, to keep the crowded chickens from going crazy, tranquillizers are put in their food and antibiotics to prevent diseases of birds. Preservatives are also added in food processing, and some of these, such as nitrites and nitrates, can be poisonous under certain conditions. Furthermore, nobody knows what the long-term effects of absorption of all these drugs will be. Perhaps the body can take care of detoxifying them all, but perhaps not. When even the penguins of Antarctica have DDT in their fat, we cannot hope to escape contamination ourselves. The Department of Agriculture of the Food and Drug Administration tries to ensure our safety, but the job is too big for it. The medical profession should be involved far more than it is, but how many think about it long enough to seek solutions? There are 75,000 acute pesticide poisonings each year in the United States. Probably there are 200 million chronic poisonings—i.e., all of us. We can only hope none of it will be fatal.

6. Food Frauds

Not long ago I was visiting relatives in America and I went to a supermarket for groceries. As I wandered about the aisles I was shaken by the sight of rows of shelves full of nonfoods. Leaving aside the tortured cereals masquerading under the name of breakfast *foods*, I saw diet colas, substitutes for coffee cream, meat substitutes, dessert fruits with sugar syrup replaced by a sweetener, and many other items including, of all things, a low-fat Chinese meal.

The idea behind this is to fool one's palate and stomach into thinking they are getting the food they like while the consumer is on a weight-losing spree or is on a restricted diet for some reason. These items are expensive; after all, it takes skill to make nothing taste like something. However, besides achieving the desired effect, the consumer may be acquiring others he does not want. The cyclamates are a case in point. It may be true, as the manufacturers claim, that one cannot absorb enough of them in the usual diet to cause cancer, as high doses have done in animals. But why take the chance? And why eat these mutilated foods at all? We do not really know what the processing is doing to them. Our knowledge of nutrition is far from complete and, in fact, some of our principles appear to be quite wrong. The old rule in medicine, "When in doubt . . . don't," applies here. We should quit mucking about with what nature provides, or confine our interference to the minimum our culture will tolerate. I would not want to eat raw wheat or meat for hygienic or esthetic reasons, but I will not eat the fantastic messes that I see in those gaudy packages. If I were still in clinical medicine I would advise my patients to leave them on the shelves.

7. Nothing Is Natural

This brings me inevitably to discussion of the organic food fads. Without going into detail I would say that, broadly speaking, I think they are good. But is anything natural any more?

The discoverer of DDT was given the Nobel Prize for his service to medicine. As it turns out, this makes about as much sense as awarding the Nobel Peace Prize to the makers of the atom bomb. Aside from its contribution to the population problem by killing malarial parasites and to agricultural problems by production of drug-resistant insects, DDT has been sprayed so enthusiastically that the whales of the Antarctic have it in their fat and penguins absorb more every time they eat a fish. The damned stuff is everywhere and its successors are almost as ubiquitous. We are assured by nutritionists that it is not harmful in the amounts present in our bodies. I do not believe them. It is concentrated in the tissues of carnivorous birds and so interferes with their reproductive processes that faulty eggs are produced. If it can do that to another carnivore, it can be doing harm to us too. We haven't yet discovered what.

We *have* discovered what another contaminant can do to us. I refer to mercury. In 1971 swordfish were banned as food in the United States because, as carnivores, they had absorbed high levels of mercury into their tissues. The mercury came from pollutants poured into the sea from our factories.

There had already been worldwide publicity over the pollution of Minamata Bay in Japan by mercury in the effluent of nearby factories. Many members of families who ate fish caught in the bay had died or suffered severe paralyses.

The problem was dramatized in the case of Mrs. N.Y., a thirty-eight-year-old over-weight Long Island housewife. She went on a reducing diet with swordfish as her principal source of energy. In nineteen months she lost forty-five pounds and gained a fine case of mercury poisoning. And this was a natural food!* In March 1972 a shipment of canned fish called flake (a pseudonym for shark) from New Zealand was seized in Australia because it had well over the maximum allowable mercury content. New Zealand

* Since writing the above I have seen a note in the *New England Journal of Medicine* that this woman has apparently had a "spontaneous remission" which brings into question the accuracy of the diagnosis of mercury poisoning since changes in the nervous system due to mercury are ordinarily irreversible. However, there is no doubt the Japanese at Minamata died of mercury pollution of fish. Nobody yet can say what are safe levels of mercury contamination. Some workers believe that chronic diseases from low levels of poisoning are passing unrecognized. Others feel that a low level of mercury poisoning may well potentiate the toxic effects of other environmental contaminants by lessening the ability of body cells e.g., in the liver, to detoxify other harmful chemicals.

is one of the most isolated countries in the world, sitting down in the South Pacific where we should expect the seas to be clean. If we want any more proof of the extent of pollution of our earth, this should provide it.

To sum up: The medical profession must accept a lot of the blame for the nutritional disasters that have blighted the twentieth century. We encouraged eating habits that produced big, healthy kids, but the habits, carried into maturity, have killed millions of men before their time. That we do not know what we are talking about is obvious in the case of the New Guinea natives who should be malnourished by our standards but continue to be hale and hearty.

We cannot be blamed for all the nutritional ills of the world. People of the West continue to eat diets they know are bad. Ignorance kills millions of children. Cultural food fads like white rice and white bread impair the health of many more. The mass-production mania is not the doctors' fault, but we must accept partial responsibility for DDT and its consequences. It is high time to rethink our theories on nutrition and get going in the right direction.

3

A Religion Called Research

1. Is Truth Where You Find It?

SAYING ANYTHING AGAINST research nowadays is like running down motherhood or blaspheming against God. Research, in fact, has become a religion, with its high priests, its acolytes, its prestigious trappings and, unfortunately, its zealotry and bigotry. Like most religions, it has its good points, but, it must be stated, some of its idols have feet of clay.

The first commandment of research is "Thou shalt search for truth." This is fine except that the second commandment is "Wherever truth may lead, there shalt thou go nor stop to consider why." The outstanding example of this, of course, is the search for atomic energy and the resultant atomic and hydrogen bombs with their threat of annihilation of life. But the medical profession is as short-sighted as any other. When to the doctors' blurred vision has been added the chronic myopia of politicians the results have been catastrophic. I have spoken of that in Chapter 1 and will again in Chapters 12 and 13. Here I want to point to other misdirections.

2. The Cuckoo's Egg in the Teacherbird's Nest

In the early 1920s a Canadian general practitioner called Frederick Banting and a young medical student, Charles Best, working in cramped quarters at the University of Toronto, discovered insulin. Banting never went back to his practice and Best became a physiologist after he graduated. Both were my teachers when, in the Banting Institute in the early 1930s, I took my B.A. in Biological and Medical Sciences. They had been awarded the Nobel Prize for their efforts. In those early days researchers were more likely to be part-time, and teaching or medical practice was how they earned their living. Today things have changed. The tiny egg of research hatched out a bird that grew and grew until today it is in danger of taking over the teacherbird's nest.

Some institutions today are purely for research and many medical and paramedical personnel are employed there full-time. In other cases medical schools have large and expensive research programs led by professors who may spend very little time teaching. In fact, it is a common complaint that undergraduates are fobbed off with instructors who are postgraduate students working toward a higher qualification. Most of these, too, are involved in the service of the god, so teaching tends to suffer. Worse still, the professors are picked for their research ability and the prestige (second only to the football team) that follows their discoveries. As I learned years ago, many of them couldn't teach worth a damn, either because they were unable to come down to our basic level or because they were unskillful in the teacher's art.

There is a moderate reversion of feeling about this nowadays. Professors are beginning once more to be valued for what they can teach. The days of Sir William Osler may yet come back.

3. Sophistication Requires Subsidization

As research has grown and as equipment has become increasingly sophisticated and therefore extremely expensive, the universities have found themselves unable to finance their research programs. Some have had support from various foundations, but in the United States the greater part of the money has come from government agencies.

In early 1971 the Department of Health, Education and Welfare budgeted $68,800 million dollars for the year beginning July 1. Of this amount $1,283 million was for biomedical research. The National Institutes of Health were to get $1,890 million. These astounding sums are not always the result of demands by the medical profession. Sometimes they are evidence of the prevalent American attitude that you can have anything you want if you just pay enough.

The previous year Elliot L. Richardson, Secretary of HEW, went before the Senate to ask that they delete some of the funds they had appropriated—e.g., an extra $74 million to expand research in cancer and genetics. He said that spending this money would cut into a program for training doctors and suggested that medical services rated priority over research in view of the doctor shortage. According to the *American Medical News* of August 24, 1970, Senator Warren G. Magnuson replied, "Why can't we have both doctors and research? I'm for putting more money into cancer research. When you've got a good thing you should spend more on it."

Later Richardson commented, "I'm up against the Washington syndrome. This is the simple-minded theory that social problems will just disappear if you throw enough dollars and statute books at them."

Subsidization leads to other problems. It is a matter of prestige for a university to have a big and active research program. Also if one can get grants for research one can hire doctors and other scientists anxious to get their names on some publications and these people can often be used part-time for teaching. The whole thing is self-perpetuating. Support depends on publications, which depend on research, which depends on more support. This may lead to good work, but all too often it leads to inferior research and "feather-bedding" as harried professors strive to keep themselves and their departments at the top of the struggling hierarchy in the academic world.

I remember my own experience when I returned from the Army to complete my training in pathology. The professor was an old friend and anxious to help me get started again after my years in the service, away from pathology.

"You'll be rusty," he said, "but I think I've got the job for you. I'll make you a Teaching Fellow and you can demonstrate to the medical students. It shouldn't be too hard to keep one class ahead of them while you relearn what you've forgotten. But you'll have to do some research."

"Why is that?" I asked. "I'm not the research type."

"The only way I can hire you is against a research grant I've managed to get. I'll give you a project."

And so I spent a year trying to duplicate the findings of a famous researcher on thyroids. It convinced me he was quite wrong, which didn't raise my opinion of his methods or conclusions, but did give me an insight into the extremely wasteful world of research with its innumerable dreary repetitions of often worthless work. The waste is likely to continue as long as people like Senator Magnuson think that they can buy brains and ensure results with money. As long ago as 1962 Dr. Paul Weiss warned that the tidal wave of today's scientific work may bury a true scientific discovery under the bulk of haphazard probing in many directions. Very few people seem to have listened.

4. Results or Rubbish?

One of the peculiarities of modern man is his belief in "facts." Take an opinion, make it respectable with numbers, graphs and charts and it becomes truth. Even scientists are not immune. Until Einstein came along and looked at things from a different viewpoint, they were quite sure that light traveled in a straight line. From where they stood, that was fact. So it is with research in medicine. Yesterday's facts are often today's fiction.

I was taught that life came in cellular packets of definite shape and usually with a nucleus in them. The exception was bacteria, but they at least had a definite cell wall, or so we thought until someone discovered that they could be L-forms lacking a normal rigid structure. Then came viruses which could enter a cell and disappear completely as they became part of the structure. Even worse, it was possible to strip off the outer parts of viruses and recombine them with different centers and yet the darned things still acted as if they were alive. So much for the facts of my youth!

Today I make my living as a histopathologist. I examine diseased tissues and make a diagnosis. This is especially important in oncology, the study of tumors. I tell the surgeon if the growth he wants to remove is benign or malignant. I give it a name which I have learned through years of training and experience and, having been pigeon-holed, the tumor is then classified in a complicated registry and one more ''fact'' is added to the billions of statistics on the incidence of tumors in various people in various parts of the world. But is this truth?

A few years ago some veterinarian isolated one of those pesky viruses from a tumor in an animal. He injected it into other animals and the results were shattering. The virus could, and did, produce tumors of several different kinds. So, after years of learning the differences, it appears that they are merely various manifestations of the work of a virus. I had suspected this myself, having seen some tumors grow and spread and, on entering different tissues, change their cellular appearances. Fortunately, these tumors do have different growth characteristics and different responses to available treatments, so the surgeon still wants me to tell him what kind of cancer he is dealing with. Otherwise I'd be out of a job. I will be, the day some bright chap discovers a vaccine for these viruses and cancer becomes history.

From what I have said above, it can be seen that much of the research into the classification of tumors will be reduced to rubbish if we discover the underlying cause of these appearances. Like a woman dressed for bed or for a banquet, what is underneath is the same.

Another place where results may be rubbish is in clinical studies. For at least fifty years arguments have raged over just how much surgery should be done in cancer of the breast. Procedures were fairly simple until techniques were perfected. Then radical mastectomy, with widespread removal of skin, breast, chest muscle and lymph glands, was advocated, with or without radiation therapy. Later cytotoxic drugs were added. The results in terms of mortality were not all that much better and the advocates of simpler procedures became vociferous again. Today each clinic has its own ideas on what to do for best results. Since the cancers vary in rate of growth and spread and patients vary in natural resistance, the possible combinations of treatment are numerous and estimating their worth would drive even an IBM statistician to drink and his computer to a short circuit. Judging by the results, there is no clear answer yet and so the research and the arguments continue.

The problem gets worse when doctors, looking into the same eyes, listening to the same hearts, examining the same laboratory results, come up with different opinions. This is obvious in recent battles over the proper treatment of diabetics, where some of the drugs have been suspected of increasing the death rate in diabetics with heart trouble. Other researchers deny that this is so, and the drug houses, with millions of dollars depending on the issue, put out as much propaganda as the cigarette manufacturers do over lung cancer. The controversy over whether or not the Pill causes thrombophlebitis is another example. How much of what was written was research . . . and how much rubbish?

The thalidomide disaster of ten years ago is a prime example of rubbishy research. I was present at the first autopsy of a case in Canada, a horribly deformed child that, fortunately, was born dead. The "facts" presented seemed to show that the drug was safe, and so it may be, except for unborn children. Today we are having a scare over hexachlorophene, which has been used by millions as a deodorant in soap. Now it appears it can cause brain damage in newborn children washed with it. How many more statistically safe products are in the same category? Worse still, how much of the research on single drugs is applicable when they are used in willful or unintended combinations with other newly-researched products? One of these days we could kill ourselves this way.

5. The Elephant Gives Birth to a Mouse

With over half the deaths and much of the illness in the civilized world ascribed to the effects of arteriosclerosis, as seen in heart attacks and strokes, it is understandable that millions of dollars and man-hours are being spent on research into causes and cures. Millions more are spent on treatment. What is the result?

So far nobody has come up with a cure, only with palliatives ranging from heart operations, transplants, pacemakers, emergency-care units to antihypertensives, cholesterol-lowering diets and so on. This looks like a tremendous effort, and it is, but what is the result? People are still getting sick and dying with the disease. They are dying younger too. In terms of results, lowering of morbidity and mortality, the elephant has labored and delivered a mouse.

This is not true of lung cancer, where statistical methods have demonstrated the cause and shown the way to prevention, if only we will take it. Yet vast efforts are still directed to cure of the condition by mutilating operations and sickening cytotoxic drugs because people will not listen. Research in these directions is largely rubbish. It would not be necessary if we enforced prevention, made cigarette manufacturers criminally liable for the effects of their product, gave them and the automobile manufacturers an unbreakable deadline by which to produce a harmless product.

6. The Do-It-Yourself Craze

One of the sacred shibboleths of medicine is that everybody should do research. Young doctors engaged in postgraduate training are especially subjected to pressure to produce something worthwhile. At medical meetings all over the world papers are read on investigations undertaken by various individuals into diseases present in their own hospitals and communities. As one eminent zealot said in Britain last year, "Any hospital where there is no research is decadent." Somewhere in his successful career he had forgotten that hospitals are primarily for treating patients, not for using them as guinea pigs.

In a recent issue of *Military Medicine* the editorial writer stated, "Inherent then in our mission of rendering highest quality medical care is an aggressive and responsive military medical research and development program *not just in the problems unique to the Armed Forces but to those areas of patient care of all categories*." [Italics mine.] Times have not changed. Years ago the inspectors came to one of the largest U.S. Armed Forces hospitals, where I happened to be serving, to look into the way it was being run. At that time there was a very vigorous clinical research program under way. When the inspectors left I asked one of the administrators what they had said. He knew I was fed up with all the medical meetings that kept me from getting on with my work.

He grinned at me. "They reported that an undue amount of time was being spent on nonpatient activities, and that if doctors would pay more attention to their clinical duties instead of to research and meetings, there would be fewer complaints from patients."

The drive to do research can lead to unfortunate complications, as in the recent outcries over the use of unsuspecting patients for implanting cancer cells. The fact that the patients were incurable does not excuse the concealment. There are other unfortunate results. I remember in one hospital a very keen internist who used to order numerous laboratory tests in the days before the multichannel autoanalyzers. One day my chief technician came to me quite upset because he was having to take numerous blood samples from an old lady dying with cancer. She had poor veins and was also having numerous intravenous medications. When I remonstrated with the doctor in charge, he said, "We need these tests. We don't know enough about electrolyte and other chemical imbalances in old people who are seriously ill. I'm doing research on them."

"But she's had enough," I protested. "Too many needles."

"I must know the electrolyte levels," he maintained. "I'm keeping her alive with these treatments."

"You aren't treating her," I said. "You're titrating her."

A few days later the old lady rebelled and refused to have any more injections and infusions. The doctor came to see her and insisted she continue her treatment.

"You leave me alone," she said. "I know I'm dying and I want to do it in peace and dignity."

Since then I have worked in hospitals where no research was done. The medical care was as good as anywhere else. Medical leaders seem to have forgotten the great men of the past who worked at the bedside. Each case was a problem to be studied and solved (research of a sort), but compassion and understanding of the patient's emotional needs were not neglected. He never became a statistic.

It is not necessary to do formal research to be a good doctor, and the sooner the high priests learn this, the less wasteful of money and manpower they will be. They might also learn something they have forgotten: It is still possible to make pertinent observations about disease in the course of one's daily duties. I never did research in my five years in Kenya, although research teams were all around me and were continually coming and going from Europe and America. I was the routine pathologist who kept things going. Nevertheless, in that five years I reported on one small disease new to science; reported the presence in East Africa of a disease called tumoral calcinosis that was not uncommon but had been hiding under the disguise of several other conditions (this led to its recognition in at least two other countries); reported for the first time the occurrence in Kenya of several fungus and parasitic conditions and made some pertinent remarks, now being confirmed, on relationships between certain tumors. Not one day was spent on formal research, but I don't believe I am decadent yet.

7. The Paper Tidal Wave

Years ago in the *Canadian Medical Association Journal* someone made a suggestion that all doctors, even in general practice, should do research and write papers about it.

"What do you think about that?" a friend asked me.

"My God," I groaned, "who could possibly read all that crap? It would take enough paper to deforest half of British Columbia. However, as a shareholder in B.C. Pulp and Paper, I'll get rich."

I do not recall the exact figures, but I believe there are about 2,200 biomedical periodicals now being published. There are free magazines, supported by advertising, which specialize in extracts of supposedly important papers from other journals, in the style of *Reader's Digest*. Even this is too much, and I know of one publication that consists entirely of the headings and titles of other medical magazines' articles from which the reader is supposed to pick out those that might interest him.

In the book world more and more hardback and expensive tomes on every conceivable aspect of medicine flood the market. Many are poorly written and horribly dull, but they do contain millions of facts, some of which are useful if they can be found among the masses of junk. The result of this tidal wave is that we are drowned in a sea of knowledge and frustrated by knowing that we will never find in it many of the things we should know.

It has been suggested that all these articles and books should be read and condensed or extracted, with the useful knowledge filed and computerized so that it could easily be retrieved by any researcher. The trouble is that the average librarian is not a doctor and cannot decide what and when and where to file these data. And where will we find trained medical people who will sit at such a dreadful task day after day?

No, the paper deluge has to stop. It should stop at the editor's desk. It must stop at the professor's door, which will happen only when the religion called research is exposed to sane thinking.

8. Will It Sell?

The after-effects of new discoveries are often unexpected. Sometimes they are carried over into other fields, as, for example, the sensors developed to monitor body functions in astronauts which are now used in Intensive Care Units or in artificial limbs. These are discussed elsewhere. One unwanted side effect of the new biochemical discoveries is advertising.

When penicillin was discovered the advent of World War II made immediate production of vast quantities mandatory. Chemical engineers were called in to devise great vats to grow the fungus and other equipment to extract and bottle the drug. A new industry was born. Since then the drug industry has expanded enormously and with it the fierce competition for the consumer's dollar. But the doctor is the one who writes prescriptions and so a flood of advertising is directed at him. He is deluged with brand names, drowned in statistics, tumbled in a surf of abstruse biochemical terminology and cast up on the beach, battered and brainwashed, to sign for he knows not what mysterious hydrocarbon with magical properties.

That is bad enough, but the drug houses have their own research laboratories. When they find a product they think is useful—for example, another antibiotic—they get it approved as safe by the government concerned and then expend millions of dollars advertising it and trying quite openly to take business away from their competitors. This kind of research, with profit as the motive, is not always in the best interests of the sick. Drugs are rushed out to market too quickly and praised too lavishly. Once in a while, as in the case of thalidomide, disaster results. As I write this, it has just been announced that Dr. William McBride, the Australian gynecologist who first warned us of the effects of thalidomide, has found more cases of phocomelia (flipper limbs) in children born of mothers who used imipramine (tofranil) during their pregnancy. This drug is a popular antidepressant. To be fair, the manufacturers warned that it should not be used in pregnancy, but, as Dr. McBride points out, a woman may not realize she is pregnant for several months and that is the most dangerous time for the fetus.

In the burgeoning field of laboratory testing and instrumentation we are also seeing the results of the rush for profit. Big chemical companies are shouldering aside private laboratories run by pathologists and are offering batteries of tests at mass-production rates. Instrument companies are putting out a bewildering array of analyzers, assayers and computers and are offering new techniques for testing. Medicine is being mechanized in every conceivable way. With profit as the motive, it is possible to lose sight of the real needs of the patient. He can do without much of this paraphernalia, and so, if we are honest about it, we must conclude that the research involved in producing it is unnecessary.

9. The Relevance of Research

For years I have felt that much of the research being done today is too unimportant to be worthwhile except to fill medical magazines and bring the author to the attention of others, on the "publish or perish" principle. Much excellent work is done, but its relevance to medicine is doubtful. I get support for this theory from a most unexpected source, Sir Macfarlane Burnet, the Nobelist in medicine. Recently I read a quote from his book *Genes, Dreams and Realities* in which he said, "None of my juniors seem to be as worried as I am, that the contribution of laboratory science to medicine has virtually come to an end." He went on later to say, "*Almost none of modern basic research in the medical sciences has any direct or indirect bearing on the prevention of dis-*

ease or on the improvement of medical care." [Italics mine.] Sir Macfarlane is now an old man. Perhaps his judgment has been warped by the disillusionment that increasing age may bring. But if he is right. . . ?

10. Non-Statistical Significance

Medical research to most people means dealing with something concrete, something measurable by material standards. Yet if we remember that all diseases have some psychological component and that mental patients occupy over half of the hospital beds in the United States, we should be far more concerned than we are about psychiatric conditions.

Biochemical research has shown that there are measurable chemical changes in diseases such as schizophrenia and homosexuality. The success of the tranquillizers, antidepressives, stimulants, relaxants and so on have shown that mental conditions can be affected by chemical compounds. Nevertheless, there is still a tremendous gap in our knowledge of psychiatric problems—a gap that may never be closed by a drug or treatment as we now know them.

There are some very curious phenomena in medicine. Recently there has been a spate of articles on cures by acupuncture, anesthesia by acupuncture and so on, brought about by the reopening of mainland China to American visitors. It may well be that acupuncture simply alters electrical charges in the nerves affected by the needles. We already know that stimulation of larger nerves will block pain impulses from their tributaries. Perhaps hypnosis plays a part, and hypnosis itself is a most curious phenomenon, difficult to investigate. Recently it was shown that, with training, human beings can alter brain waves at will by putting themselves in the right frame of mind. The yogis of India and the lamas of Tibet are reputed to be capable of mentally controlling the "insensible" functions of the body, such as elimination, respiration, circulation, and of being able to go into a sort of hibernation by thinking about it. We have scoffed at such travelers' tales for generations. They may be true.

Think of what we could achieve by such controls over body function! Think of what we might do by conscious control of some mental functions. There are those who believe we can wish away warts. Some of them are doctors. Now, warts are caused by viruses. If we could control them by wishing—i.e., by thought control—perhaps we could learn to control cancer, which I believe is also viral in many cases, if not all. Fantastic? Perhaps so, but I can remember when radio was new and television unheard of. There may be other natural forces we have not yet discovered. God knows we need some way to control the human race before it destroys itself and the world. That is the sort of research, dangerous though it may be, that could be of the greatest significance even if it is not measurable by our slide rules.

One final thought about research: I and many other doctors have often thought we should have a moratorium on research of all kinds, medical and otherwise, and use the funds saved to put into effect what we have already learned. Dr. Morris E. Chafetz, Director of the National Institute of Alcohol Abuse and Alcoholism, told the *American Medical News* in October 1971, "One of our greatest problems related to research today is how to utilize the research findings we already have."

I think that idea was best expressed by the California farmer who was asked why he didn't study ways for making his good farm even more productive. He answered, "I got more knowin' now than I does, and until the doin' I does catches up with the knowin' I has, I can't see no reason for knowin' no more."

4

Dr. Robot

1. In the Beginning

IT MAY BE COINCIDENCE, but it seems to me that the amazing proliferation of machines in medicine was one of the responses, as tissue replacements were, to the frightening increase in the amount of heart disease. Aside from accidents, heart attacks are probably the most dramatic medical emergencies in modern times, and more frightening because we feel so helpless—there are no tourniquets or bandages to apply to wounds, no splints for twisted limbs. The doctor called to the house twenty-five years ago could do little but give a hypodermic of some pain-relieving drug, along with some coramine or adrenalin, and call for an ambulance. A few years later some brave souls ventured to slash through the chest muscles and grasp the heart itself, squeezing life-saving blood to the brain until the hospital was reached and the newly designed instruments could take over.

Today we have specially equipped ambulances with pacemakers and respirators, radio communications and other refinements designed to keep the patient alive until he reaches the inner sanctum, the new holy of holies, the Intensive Care Unit.

2. The Inner Sanctum

The Intensive Care Unit is probably the finest example of the application of engineering to medicine that has ever been seen.

Within its walls are fearsomely complicated and horrifyingly expensive gadgets that a few years ago were just a physicist's dream. I do not know what a cube interferometer is, nor an impedance plethysmograph. I have trouble saying the names, never mind knowing what they do. When I was younger, sonar was a way of detecting submarines near our convoy. Now they use ultrasonic echo-ranging, the same thing, to examine patients.

With catheters thrust down a vein into a major vessel or the heart itself, blood pressures are monitored and the blood is continuously analyzed for its gases and electrolytes. The patient is wired to electrocardiographs, electroencephalographs and pacemakers. He is attached by a tracheotomy to a respirator that breathes for him, to tubes that feed him, to dialyzers that remove the wastes from his blood. He cannot speak, he is afraid to move, he listens to the humming and beeping of Space Age instruments. In fact, he is wired like an astronaut and almost as isolated from anything familiar. He could be dead for hours and still his heart would be made to beat and his lungs to breathe. Only the straight penned line on the electroencephalograph tape would tell the truth: the spirit had gone.

The ICU has been a great success, so the enthusiasts claim. Ten years ago about 30 percent of all heart-attack patients who reached a hospital died there. Nowadays the rate has been cut to 20 percent or less. ICUs in pediatric hospitals do even better, with survival rates close to 90 percent. There are some dissenting voices. A recent study in Great Britain claimed that the survival rate of cardiac cases treated in smaller hospitals by modern methods but without most of the paraphernalia was almost as good. It was thought that the patients themselves and their relatives were happier away from the awesome array of machines which have frightened doctors too when they became patients.

When we consider that it can cost $500 per day in an ICU and in America this is often not covered by insurance, we have to sit back and wonder if perhaps we should let simpler methods be used, a calculated risk which, if it comes off, will make the future a lot pleasanter for both patient and family, who will still have some money left to live on.

The hospitals too are worried by all this mechanization. It costs them more than they charge the patients. It requires specially trained squads of doctors, nurses and assistants. It requires technicians trained to handle and repair electronic equipment, and, with all that, the machines may be both unsafe and unreliable. To quote Dr. Ian Donald from the *Medical Tribune*, December 1970, on the subject of monitoring techniques, "In fact yards and yards of tracing may be rather less important than direct clinical observation and from the patient's point of view a little intelligent human supervision may be more effective and informative."

In 1971, in Malawi, I talked to a young doctor from Wayne University who had come out to work in a medical mission. He was specializing in heart disease, but saw very little in Africa, to his surprise. I was curious about ICUs, as I had never seen a really modern one.

"What about the machines?" I asked. "Are they reliable?"

"That's one of our problems," he replied. "We did a study of hospitals in Detroit not so long ago and found that many of the machines were defective in some way or another. They were giving false results. It requires constant vigilance and frequent inspections to be sure they are working properly."

So much for our belief that the machine does not lie. Truth is not a wave of ink on a sheet of paper.

The efficacy of machines is often overrated. For example, in a recent study on tetanus, a disease now rare in the West but seen frequently in more primitive areas, it was shown that, with highly sophisticated machinery for monitoring and keeping the patient breathing, the results were little better than without such apparatus. The death rate in 20 patients treated at the United Oxford Hospitals, England, in 1938-42 was 25 percent. In 1954-58 for 32 patients the rate was 22 percent. In 1964-68 for 32 patients the rate was also 22 percent. It was stated that *most cases survived on less specialized and expensive therapy such as was available in Ghana, Africa, in 1969*. Antibiotics were not available in the first series quoted, but antiserum was.

Just to illustrate the complexity of the modern treatment, I enumerate the machines set up to treat the tetanus cases in 1964-68:

Using an arterial catheter, the blood was monitored by an electromanometer and cardiotachometer and samples were taken for blood gas pressures and biochemistry.

By venous catheters at various distances, even into the heart, the electromanometer and a cuvette densitometer were used and venous blood samples were taken for analysis.

By an airway catheter an infra-red gas analyzer measured carbon dioxide. An electrocardiograph monitored the heartbeats, using an amplifier and oscilloscope plus a cardiotachometer.

A rectal thermistor using a Wheatstone bridge and amplifier measured the temperature of the body.

The patient also had a device installed for collection of urine. When breathing was inadequate a mechanical respirator could also be used.

The cost of all this can be imagined. The results, as shown above, were no better.

There are other drawbacks. All that electrical equipment can be dangerous. Patients can receive severe shocks from faulty machines or from unintentional grounding when hooked up to the monitors. Some patients are psychologically disturbed by the equipment and the isolation from visitors which may be necessary. Any old-time GP will tell you about the need for TLC (tender loving care) handed out by nurses and family visitors. But the nurse watching a dozen beds by closed-circuit television and pulling tape out of a scanner like a Wall Street banker in a bull market hasn't much time for pillow patting. She hasn't much time to sit and chat either, and the patient doesn't get his fears explained away. The doctor too has to be careful not to look at his patient as a computer print-out or he can find that, in spite of a favorable electrolyte balance and a satisfactory electrocardiograph, the man is not doing well. In primitive societies human beings can and do still die from fear. What makes us think we are so different?

3. Hotel in a Hospital

Once out of the ICU, the patient is back in a more familiar setting, and he pays for it. Let us look at what I call the high cost of comfort, or the hotel in a hospital.

In August 1971, while on vacation in the United States, my son slashed a tendon in his hand the day before we were to leave. He was admitted to a hospital at 2:00 P.M., had his operation later that afternoon and was released to my care at 8:00 A.M. the next day to catch a plane.

The service charge for the room was $43. The use of the operating room for, I presume, less than an hour cost $75. Medicines cost $30 and the laboratory $19. Other minor charges came to $11. The surgeon did not charge me for his services.

Operating rooms, like ICUs, are full of gadgets. The hourly rental has to be high. The hospital room was semiprivate and, in my view, far more expensive than need be. There were no cheaper rooms. My son lay on an electrically controlled bed and amused himself pushing buttons to make it lift or fold up in various ways. Beside him was a telephone, and, of course, a television set flickered across the room. Toilet facilities were in a small bathroom in the suite.

Very little of this was really necessary. It may save a few seconds of the nursing aide's time not to have to adjust beds by winding a handle, but what about the patient who is supposed to be nursed in a certain position and insists on changing it by pushing a button? What about the danger of electric shock? Above all, what about the cost of such a bed and of regular maintenance? The telephone was a luxury and so was the television, although I can hear the indignant protests of popeyed TV fans about that. The fact is that, except for patients condemned to days or weeks of confinement, we could dispense with many of these services. Senator Abraham Ribicoff in a recent article said that 35 percent of the increase in hospital costs over the last few years was because of more services provided per person. We could reduce that amount by being more spartan.

In Britain patients not requiring intensive care but needing to be watched are being nursed in convalescent hospitals where special equipment is at a minimum and where the patient is expected to look after himself to some extent. The cost is much lower.

4. The Medical Man's Machines

Another area where mechanization is taking over is in the doctor's office, especially in group practices where several doctors can use the same machines and so justify the expense. Rather than send a patient to a hospital for tests, it is often possible to have them done in the office—for example, an electrocardiograph in suspected heart disease. The amount of sophistication depends to some extent on the size and wealth of the clinic concerned. It seems only a question of time until computer-assisted diagnosis becomes common. The patient will tick off answers to a questionnaire, have blood taken, possibly by a machine, be X-rayed if the computer decides it is necessary, and end his tour of the clinic where the clinical assistant or perhaps the doctor will consider the computer's diagnosis, check a few points himself and carry out the suggested treatment. The shock will come when the bill arrives, or, if Kennedy-style politicians manage to bring in total governmental medical care, when the taxpayer finds out what he owes.

The ultimate in medical men's machinery so far is the multiphasic screening laboratories of the Kaiser Permanente Medical Care Program, a prepaid group-practice scheme. The idea is to use equipment to perform multiple tests and then, by computer, separate the sick from the well. I cannot describe here all that is done, but it includes the electrocardiograph, chest X-ray, eye examination, respiratory measurements, audiometry, self-administered medical and psychological questions (355 in all) on prepunched sorting cards and finally about twenty-five separate laboratory tests of blood and urine. For older people there is also sigmoidoscopy and a gynecological examination for women. Ten days later a computer summary is printed out. The patient then sees a physician.

A study of this way of handling medical care is not yet complete, but it is considered that such procedures will raise the cost of medical care in spite of the speed of the machines. The crunch comes in tentative conclusions by observers, as follows: "There is at present, and there will continue to be in the very near future, no scientific evidence on the value of screening in terms of its ultimate benefit in reducing morbidity and mortality." The old-time Yankee would have called that buying a pig in a poke.

What a computer can do to assist the patient with an anxiety neurosis, other than advising tranquillizers, I do not know. Perhaps the engineers will be able to make one that looks and talks like the friendly old GP used to. It might work if there is another computer in town listening to all the gossip and aware of what caused the patient's problems in the first place.

One place where machinery has really run wild is the laboratory. Fortunately for old-timers like me, there is no machine that can do an autopsy or diagnose cancer on a biopsy of a breast. There is one that can screen out normal cervical smears and it may soon be good enough to print out diagnoses on abnormal ones. It is in biochemistry and, to a lesser extent, in routine hematology that the machine is replacing the technician and turning out batteries of tests infinitely faster and more accurately than was done before. But there are drawbacks.

In a recent study of automated laboratory systems the author warned that such a system does not allow savings by firing technicians. What it does do is allow technicians to perform more tests in a given time at a lower cost per test. To me this poses the question: Are more tests really necessary? I quote from Dr. D. W. Penner of Winnipeg, Canada, in the *Bulletin of the College of American Pathologists*, February 1970: "Skyrocketing costs of laboratory services are proving to be a serious drain on funds available for payment of insured medical services. In the past few years the cost of these services per insured person has increased 500 percent." Later, in April 1970, he reported, "One large clinical pathology area was unable to do anything but emergency work for a period of four days because of automated equipment failure. This was the third such failure in three months. *The great reduction in work did not seem to adversely affect patient care. Does this perhaps suggest a slight trend toward overuse because it is free?*" [Italics mine for the first sentence, his for the second.] I am quite sure it does and also suggests one more application of the law that if equipment is available, it will be used whether needed or not, and that, after Parkinson's Law, the work to fill the time available will be generated.

Another aspect of this machine madness is not generally realized. The machines report a level of chemicals and we know the so-called normal values. But there is no such thing as normal. Various methods give slightly differing ranges of normal and some people are quite different from the usual. For example, the ratio of albumen to globulin in an African's blood may be the reverse of the usual in an American. His white count may be so low that it would worry the American doctor, but it is normal for him. I myself have a blood pressure about forty points below the average (I do not say normal) white man of my age, but about the same as that in the uncivilized African. So all these measurements must be used with caution in our interpretation of disease. Measurements may also vary considerably, depending on how samples are taken; for example, keeping a tourniquet on too long will make some chemical determinations vary a great deal. The time of day and how much and what was eaten will also matter. I mention this only to show that figures can lie if not interpreted with caution.

To justify spending $50,000 or more on a multichannel analyzer, there must be enough tests to keep the machine busy. This limits it to larger hospitals or clinics. Smaller models or machines that perform one test repeatedly are on the market. They may be used in smaller institutions. All of them require constant supervision to ensure accuracy, and a certain amount of "down time" for repairs or maintenance cannot be avoided. Unless the hospital has its own generators, none of these instruments will work in a power brown-out, and power shortages are likely to become a real headache in the very near future, if we are to believe recent reports.

Hours of argument and reams of statistics have been used in trying to decide whether it is cheaper and better to do all the tests every time the patient's blood is taken (as the multichannel analyzer does) or, after an initial "base-line" of tests is obtained, to select a few tests which seem to be helpful in making the diagnosis or watching the course of the disease. The way Americans move about these days, it will require computer link-ups all over the country if we are to know in California what were the clinical and laboratory findings in Mr. John Doe ten years ago in a New York hospital. Like the controversy on credit ratings, this could bring legal headaches, especially if there were some embarrassing tests in the patient's past history. What will happen to a doctor in future who ignores the diagnosis given him by a computer and is later involved in a malpractice suit is an interesting speculation.

The problem of how much laboratory work to do may sometimes be solved quite outside medical considerations. As I mention in Chapter 10, many procedures that are not really necessary are done as a hedge against a future malpractice suit. Juries believe in "facts," and batteries of tests are impressive evidence of a doctor's proficiency and modernity.

5. Mechanical Man

Mechanization does have a bright side. It has made life infinitely better for paraplegics, who can now get out of hospitals. It has provided wonderful artificial limbs with built-in servomechanisms for children deformed by thalidomide. It may supply sonar range-finding for the blind, on the same principle used by bats to fly in the dark. Eventually it may be possible to hook up prostheses to the ends of amputated nerves and use them almost like real limbs. For these and other devices we should be thankful.

Another type of mechanical man becoming increasingly common is the one with an artificial pacemaker for his heart. In many survivors from heart attacks the nervous mechanism that keeps the heart beating regularly is so badly damaged that control of the contractions is unreliable and the patient could die at any moment if the nervous stimulus puts the heart into what is called fibrillation or flutter—i.e., a series of rapid beats that do not pump the blood properly. To prevent this, our surgeons install pacemakers, formerly outside the chest but now hidden under the skin, and these keep the heart beating at the proper rate. At least, that is the theory. However, we are now running into that plague of the production line, faulty assembly.

In April 1972 nearly five hundred pacemakers manufactured by General Electric were suspected of being defective when it was found that some of them were speeding up heartbeats by as much as 20 per minute (the average heart beats about 72 per minute). One could paraphrase Ralph Nader and say they were unsafe at any speed. The company offered to pay all costs of the surgery required to replace the machines, much as General Motors replaces defective parts. It is a pity the general manager and his executives could not experience some of the pain of the operation as well. They might check their equipment more carefully from now on.

6. Throw It Away

A spin-off from all this mechanization which is supposed to save time and money is disposability. It is a facet of our civilization in other fields, as beer drinkers and other can users know. To eliminate dishwashing and sterilizing, most of the minor pieces of equipment are used once and thrown away. This is supposed to be more efficient and safer. The latter is open to doubt.

Sometimes the packaging of supposedly sterile disposable syringes and so on is defective. The efficiency I will not dispute. The cost is high and, of course, eventually is passed on to the consumer. Prepackaged kits of all kinds have been designed so that almost anyone can do what used to be a skillful technician's job. They include equipment such as test tubes and pipettes as well as chemicals, and all are thrown away after use. They cost money, just as TV dinners do.

One reason for making these kits is that quick results may be sent to the clinician to enable him to make quick decisions and treat the patient and get him out of the hospital as soon as possible. However, until the day comes when hospital beds are on an assembly line and the patient falls off, cured, into his car, I am not convinced that all this haste is useful. After all, if the doctor is at a ball game and the laboratory results sit in his pigeonhole, it does not matter that they reached there an hour earlier. He will get to them in his own good time. And with prepaid medical care Mrs. Jones isn't going to be shunted out of her nice bed of convalescence a day early to go back to a houseful of howling kids —not if she can help it. Perhaps I am being a bit unkind to make the point, but we are not machines and do not work like them.

7. The Neglected Computer: Man

Those of us who have lived and worked out on the edge of the world know how much of all this mechanization is luxury. It is possible to run a good medical service with one tenth of the machinery at one tenth the cost. If it were not, most of the world's people would have no medical care. The shortages of medical personnel and equipment are bad enough, even in America, to make us pause and wonder: Is there not a simpler way to do things?

In the fashionable jargon of mechanical medicine we talk of measuring various parameters. For example, the Autoanalyzer SMA 12 measures twelve parameters—i.e., twelve different chemical components of blood. The electrocardiograph used to have three leads. It now measures about thirteen electrical waves referable to different areas of the heart. Today's young doctor, up to his ears in technology, can interpret many of these measurements, but in the process of learning this he has had to neglect the skills his father had in the use of the five-parameter computer, the five senses of man: sight, hearing, smell, taste and touch.

The human computer is still the most complicated information-collecting and -correlating system on earth. The five senses, used as I have seen experienced older clinicians use them, coupled with searching questions in taking the history, will make observations with accuracy and discrimination and come up with diagnoses that are correct in the majority of cases. Add a few simple aids such as the stethoscope and ophthalmoscope and most of medical diagnosis is covered. The other expensive tests and procedures are frequently only confirmatory. They are very nice to have, if one can afford them.

The cost of the human machine is included in the doctor's bill, regardless of what he does. It should not be neglected in favor of mechanical methods. It possesses, too, a quality that cannot be built into any other machine, the quality of mercy, of compassion, of sympathy. Emotions are not measurable in the material sense, but, properly used, they may do more for a patient than anything else.

When we consider that all illness has some psychological content which in many cases is the major factor, it becomes obvious that processing people through an assembly line of machines is not the answer. Unless we mutate into emotionless imitations of man or become brainwashed into robots at the order of some future dictator, we will always need TLC in large doses, at frequent intervals. That is where the machine stops and man takes over.

8. Have we Gone Too Far?

The ICU has reduced mortality in heart attacks by perhaps 10 to 15 percent. It has increased the cost of treatment by 400 to

500 percent, although inflation must take some of the blame. Ours is a democratic and increasingly socialized society. Nobody can be denied the use of the ICU simply because he cannot afford to pay for it. Therefore, as the editors of *Newsweek* put it on May 24, 1971, "the day is not far off for ICU patients when someone will have to decide, chiefly on the basis of the cost involved, which patients shall be given a chance to live—and which shall be condemned to die."

Can we afford so many mechanical methods? Can we afford hospitals like hotels? Do we need all those laboratory tests? I believe the answer is no. Much of mechanical medicine is misdirected. We must find a better way.

5

The Doctor Shortage — Fact or Fallacy?

1. The Situation

SOMEONE ONCE SAID ABOUT POLITICS, "If you tell a lie loud enough and long enough, eventually it will be believed." To those of us living in outposts of the world like New Guinea the cry of "doctor shortage" in the United States is such a lie. It depends on what you are used to. My wife told me once she simply could not manage without a refrigerator-freezer. My mother was happy to go from icebox to a tiny "fridge." My grandmother had a cool cellar dug into the ground under the trees. She did not live long enough to know about, and therefore want, these things.

The immediate reaction to what I have just said is to snort, "We don't live like your grandmother either." More's the pity, I say, and refer you to Chapter 12. But the point has some validity. Let us try to see how much.

In 1970 the United States was said to have 166 physicians for every 100,000 persons. This is a marked increase from the level of 149 in 1959 and 153 in 1966. It varies with the states, with Alabama having about 83 per 100,000. The American rate is one of the highest in the world. Politicians have made comparisons with other nations such as the Swedish and the New Zealanders, revealing that we have a higher infant mortality and that Americans, especially males, do not live as long as they do. This is supposed to prove that we do not have enough doctors to care for us. But if we take away the Negro, the Latin American, and the poor whites—i.e., if we compare Americans on the same economic level as the Swedes, who have no race problems and no real poverty—the figures are much closer.

Aside from such comparisons, thc infant mortality rate in the United States is 20 percent less in 1972 than it was in 1965. If there is a doctor shortage, it appears to have benefited the children. Also the age-adjusted death rate for all Americans has dropped from 9.0 per thousand in 1947 to 7.3 in 1967. This is a good record. It would be a lot better if Americans would eat less, exercise more, quit smoking and drive only when sober. One can hardly blame the doctor shortage for those deaths.

2. Maldistribution—the Real Problem

Compared with most of the world, the problem in the United States is not a true shortage but a maldistribution of doctors. In every country in the world, even where medicine is socialized, the distribution of doctors is uneven. Some of this is unavoidable. For instance, one cannot have a good medical school without a concentration of teachers plus a large hospital group with more staff to help in the teaching as well as care for the patients who provide the cases for students to study. On the other hand, the distribution can be wasteful. According to Carl M. Cobb in the *Saturday Review* of August 22, 1970, of 318,000 living Americans with M.D. after their names only 203,000 are actually treating patients. Others are retired, in training, in administrative posts, in full-time teaching or research, or in positions not involved with the dispensing of medical care. This is not a true bill, as many doctors in training are working with patients, and so are teachers. Nevertheless, one wonders how much of this diversion is really necessary.

Where free movement is allowed, it is axiomatic that any skilled man will gravitate to where he can ply his trade and get the most return for his efforts. Doctors are the same. They concentrate where patients are plentiful, close together and able to pay. They want to be near hospitals and near their fellow physicians. They want good homes for their families and schools for their children. The result is a high proportion of doctors in wealthy areas of cities, especially in the more salubrious climates, and a dearth in the slums and unpleasant rural areas.

In certain parts of New York the ratio of doctors to people is approximately one to 30,000 or about the national average in Kenya. This is quite understandable. Most doctors are not missionaries, and black doctors also want to live in an environment where their wives are safe in the streets and their kids can get a decent education. They also want to be paid for what they do. In many rural areas doctors are also scarce. The distances they have to travel, the paucity of patients and the cultural and scientific isolation are reasons enough to keep them away.

3. The Jack-of-All-Trades Is Gone

Another cause of shortage is specialization. Whereas in the old days seven out of ten doctors might be general practitioners, today the ratio is reversed. This means that finding someone to take care of ordinary complaints is much harder than it was. I might say the same of tradesmen with their restrictive union practices, but, of course, that's different!

A third and probably the main reason for the shortage is overuse and misuse of doctors. With insurance plans enabling all sorts of people to get cheap rates for medical attention, the demands on the doctor's services have gone beyond all reason. My own experiences in British Columbia after the war convinced me of this. I found the same thing years later when I was in charge of the Outpatient Clinic in one of the U.S. Army's largest hospitals. There was blatant overuse of medical services.

I can think of another possible reason for the doctor shortage: the knowledge explosion. It takes more doctors to apply all the knowledge in the form of more complicated examinations, tests, treatments and so on. As long as people are conditioned to demand these services, and as long as doctors are sued for malpractice on the grounds of neglecting to use them, this situation will continue.

4. They Really are Hurting

There is no doubt whatever about the doctor shortage in the undeveloped world. It is real, and it is critical for many reasons. Millions of people are born and die without ever seeing a doctor. Millions more go to witch doctors, herbalists, faith healers and just plain quacks. Where there is a government medical service, millions go to dispensaries staffed by overworked and under-educated clinical assistants. The doctor, if there is one, will be at district headquarters, miles away. Mission hospitals help somewhat, but the difficulties of providing even basic medical care are awesome and getting worse.

From my own experience as a pathologist let me give you some examples. I arrived in Kenya six weeks after independence, in January 1964. The population was then estimated at 10 million, and I was the only pathologist in government service who held a postgraduate degree. Even in 1971 there were less than a dozen pathologists in or out of government. In Sarawak, with about 900,000 people, I was the only specialist pathologist in 1969. Today there is none. In Malawi, for 4.5 million people there is one pathologist. In Papua New Guinea, including the new medical school, there are five for 2.5 million people and when two left there were no replacements in sight.

The World Health Organization estimates that one pathologist per 100,000 people is a good goal to try for. In the directory of the College of American Pathologists for 1971 the three areas of New York City, Brooklyn and the Bronx had a total of 161 pathologists listed as members of the college. Not included were academic pathologists who may not be members but who work as specialists at least part of the time with patients. If these three boroughs contain 10 million people, then there is one pathologist for about 60,000 people. That shows us who is short of help.

In other medical specialties the situation is similar. In Kenya the doctor-patient ratio averages one to 30,000—better in the cities and much worse in the country. In Papua New Guinea recently the ratio of all listed doctors to patients was about one to 8,000 which is an excellent ratio for an undeveloped country. In the United States it averages about one to 750, more or less, depending on various calculations.

5. Too Many Doctors

In some parts of the world there is a surplus of doctors. Israel, for instance, has one to about 400 or 500 people. This is an artificial situation due to the emigration of Jews, many highly educated, from other lands. Some of them have been lent to other countries—e.g., the eye-diseases unit in Malawi is staffed by Israelis.

In the Philippines many doctors are working as clerks or taxi drivers or in business. Here the problem is twofold. Most of them want to work in the cities, and in Manila, for example, there are far too many doctors. The government pays very small salaries to those who work in rural areas and few educated men will tolerate the resulting low standard of living. Thus we have the spectacle of a country with poor medical services in the midst of a doctor surplus. Those doctors who can, emigrate to another country with better pay and living conditions. Recently the Papua New Guinea government has been looking into employing some of these Filipinos. They would cost less and probably be easier to recruit than Australians or other Europeans.

6. The Team Concept, or Old Plays in a New Game

It is one of the privileges of growing old to be able to say, "Yes, it is quite an idea, but it was tried years ago." Certainly, as regards the recent enthusiasm for having assistants to take some of the work off the American doctor, I have seen it before in India, Formosa, Kenya, Malawi and New Guinea. Note that these are either impoverished or undeveloped countries. They adopted their plans because of acute doctor shortages. We might learn from their experiences.

Thirty years ago, when I transferred from the Royal Canadian Army Medical Corps to the Indian Medical Service, I learned that not all doctors were doctors. We had in our units what were called Viceroy's commissioned officers, roughly comparable to the American warrant officer. These men, with lesser educational qualifications to begin with, had had four years of training in medicine and had then been given a license to practice. In the Army they were supervised by fully qualified physicians, but in civilian life they set up their own offices. Some were efficient, some were not; some were brashly confident, others stayed within their limitations. In other words, they acted like doctors anywhere.

In Formosa, with the Chinese Nationalist Army, I saw the same thing. Here, however, there were far fewer well-qualified physicians, and the licentiates took over much more of the duties. The results, judged by what I saw during the Quemoy-Matsu fighting in 1958, were definitely inferior by American standards. This brings me to a "new idea," the use of corpsmen trained in Vietnam as doctors' assistants.

Years ago a surgeon told me that any first-class carpenter could be trained to perform an operation. In fact, at the battle of Cassino I watched the chief assistant (he really *had* been a carpenter) skillfully clean and repair wounds of the abdomen and limbs while the exhausted surgeon took time off for a rest and a smoke. But nimble fingers are not enough. What makes a good surgeon is the ability to arrive at a diagnosis, the knowledge of when to operate and how to manage the post-operative care. The actual operation is only part of the successful management of a patient. This is where the weaknesses of quickie courses show up.

In my view, as long as assistants of any kind are adequately supervised they can be very useful. If in the exhausting routine of today's medicine we slough off too many of our responsibilities to assistants, then the quality of medical care is likely to suffer.

Assistants, being human, are ambitious. We see that today in the continuing fight between medical technicians and pathologists. Once upon a time the technicians were assistants, under medical supervision. Today they, and recently some of the big drug companies, are setting up independent laboratories. When the College of American Pathologists tried to stop this, the Justice Department brought the College into court as being "in restraint of trade."

When lawyers can equate a part of the medical profession with being a trade, it is time we look where we are going. Others of our team of assistants, and we too, could end up in labor unions. If we do, then medicine, at least in its moral and ethical aspects, will have deteriorated.

One aspect of the assistant boom needs to be looked at very critically. Empires tend to grow, and American empires are worse than most. The U.S. Army, for example, needs at least 15 men behind the rifleman on the line to keep him fighting. The Russians need about 4 and their army is first class. In the medical field, in the United States in 1900 the number of support personnel for each physician was one. Today it is 13 and by 1975 it is estimated it will be 20. If we go on at that rate, everyone will be a doctor's helper in the next century. By contrast, the Russian system is much more austere. I have no exact figures, but a pathologist who visited the U.S.S.R. in 1970 reported that laboratories were about twenty-five years behind us in methods and staffing. Judging by reports from the Russian-built and -staffed hospital we had in

Kenya in 1968, I would say that is a fair estimate. Yet the medical services in Russia seem adequate to keep the citizens in good health.

7. Will Mrs. Consumer Accept Brand X?

If the complexifiers have their way (and in America they seem to outnumber the simplifiers) we will have a double hierarchy in medicine. We will have doctors of medicine trained in all grades from the family practitioner to the cardiac surgeon. Below them will be an ever increasing organization of paramedical people. There will be nurses of various grades and specialties, midwives, laboratory technologists, technicians and technical assistants, doctor's assistants, nurse's aides, clinical psychologists, various therapists, social workers and so on. And all of them, from the lowliest to the highest, will be scrabbling for more pay, more status, more power.

When Mrs. Consumer gets sick she will probably go to a group clinic, see several of these assistants, perhaps several doctors, and then, if sick enough, go through a somewhat similar process in a hospital. It may be more efficient, but it will be more impersonal and probably more frightening. Mrs. Consumer will probably not like it, but, to be fair to the medical profession, she asked for it. When she started demanding all sorts of services and shopping around for doctors like bargains in a supermarket, she lost the personal touch, just as she lost it when the corner butcher went bankrupt.

8. The Idiot Savant

One of the disturbing aspects of the explosion of knowledge is the necessity for ultraspecialization. Take my field of pathology for example. The January 1972 *Bulletin of the Royal College of Pathologists* (of Great Britain) on "Training of Medical Graduates in Pathology'' splits pathology into five major fields: chemical pathology, hematology, immunology, medical microbiology, morbid anatomy and histopathology. Thirty years ago one pathologist might have covered them all.

My own sub-specialty of morbid anatomy and histopathology (or anatomical pathology, to use American terminology) is now further divided into exfoliative cytology, histopathology (or surgical pathology), forensic pathology (which spills over into toxicology), histochemistry and electron microscopy.

Histopathology, in larger centers, can also be broken down into full-time sub-sub-specialties such as gynecological, pediatric, orthopedic and neurological pathology. There is some overlapping, of course, but the above illustrates what has happened in only one small area of medicine. Similar sub-specialization is occurring in other branches, and entirely new disciplines such as biophysics, nuclear medicine, computer techniques and so on have sprung up. The result, to quote the old saw, is that these people ''know more and more about less and less until they know everything about nothing.''

With so many people engaged full-time in such diverse branches of medicine, more doctors are needed. Also communication between them is increasingly difficult. The specialist studying the aerodynamics of breathing, for example, will be out of touch with the electron microscopist working on the mitochondria of a brain cell. Who will coordinate all this? Who, in other words, will be able to see the woods instead of individual trees? This, it seems to me, is one of the major problems facing medicine today. Our art is sadly fragmented. Can it be made into a cohesive, understandable whole?

Today no one man can know all of a sub-branch of pathology, to say nothing of surgery or other branches. The polymath is gone, but do we have to end up with dozens of ''idiot savants''—i.e., people so specialized as to be ignorant of any other knowledge? We need a few of them in special centers, of course, but it is wasteful of medical manpower to have many, as we have today.

It might be better to leave much of the exotic lore in the research laboratories and universities, and concentrate our medical training on the "whole man." By this I mean studying man in relation to his environment, man's mental and psychological problems and, in adequate but not excessive detail (for all but specialists), man's physical diseases. This would turn out doctors who could take care of 99 percent of our ailments. It might result in cheaper medical care except for one thing: It takes time to listen to people, something most doctors cannot do enough because a doctor's time is expensive. Perhaps here is the place for paramedical people. In fact, there is already a trend toward having sympathetic and worldly-wise counsellors, not necessarily (and some doctors say not at all) with medical or psychological training, available to listen. Ministers of various religions are also coming back into prominence in such work, another indication that medicine has been going the wrong way as it follows the path of pure materialistic science.

9. Regimentation the Solution?

As I mentioned previously, various attempts have been made to correct maldistribution of doctors. In the United States substituting service in depressed areas for military service is one proposal. In New Zealand doctors are subsidized by government to practice in depressed native settlements. In Saskatchewan some years ago the socialist government brought in legislation giving it power to order doctors to practice wherever the politicians wanted. The result was one of the first doctors' strikes in the world. The politicians capitulated and then called an election, confident that the people would be angry with the medical profession. To a man the socialists lost their seats, and a new government took over. For once people seemed to realize that regimentation of one profession could lead to loss of freedom for all.

Canada seems to have had its share of politicians who attempt to force medicine in their direction. In 1971 it was the Minister of Health of Quebec at war with the medical specialists. Recently it has been the government of British Columbia with its provincial medical plan which would give it power to prevent doctors practicing where they will. In Great Britain, where medicine is already highly socialized, dissatisfaction is continuous and the costs, hidden in confiscating taxes, are appallingly high. The battle is already in progress in the United States, with Senator Edward Kennedy and his cronies the leading exponents of welfare-statism. One wonders whether he and his fellow politicians would endure restrictions on their political and business practices similar to those they urge on the medical profession.

Here, I feel, is the crux of the matter. In a true democracy, such as the United States is supposed to be, how can the "right to medical care" so loudly proclaimed by so many, but not to be found in the Constitution, be allowed to interfere with the liberty of doctors, as individuals, to live and work anywhere, which *is* in the Constitution. The day I am forced by law to practice medicine in one place, in one organization and no other, is the day I shall insist that everyone else, in whatever walk of life, shall march in lock-step with me to our imprisonment. That day may come, if the direction of medicine is not changed.

6

Medical Education — Where Is It Going?

1. Instant Doctors

THE CONTINUING OUTCRY about the supposed doctor shortage in the United States has helped to focus attention on medical education. Not since the Flexner Report, which shook up American medical schools in 1910, has there been so much discussion. New medical schools are being founded and each one has its own idea on how doctors should be trained and in what direction their training should lead them. The same confusion extends to the training of paramedical personnel.

In 1971 there were 108 medical schools in the United States. Five of them had just opened. Eight more were expected to open in 1972. The total enrollment for 1970-71 was 40,487, an increase of 2,818 over the previous year. Twelve thousand five hundred began their studies in September 1971, an increase of about 40 percent over the 1965 figures and a much greater percentage rise than the population increase for the same period.

In 1970, 8,367 doctors were graduated. But a doctor's education does not end there. Almost all go on for postgraduate hospital practice, and for some specialties that could mean another five years. With all sorts of people screaming about inadequate medical care in the United States, which makes citizens of the undeveloped world think of them as rich spoiled brats, those in positions of power, both political and medical, have been searching for solutions. One partial solution is delegation of some responsibility to paramedical personnel. Another is to shorten the medical course.

It was announced in 1971 that twenty-five U.S. medical schools will now award the M.D. in less than four years from the student's date of entry. Most have dropped the course to three years. There is also some agitation to shorten pre-medical studies, and one way would be to go for twelve months of the year instead of having a long summer vacation. That would be fine except that the students still count on making a bit of cash in summer. Perhaps they could all be subsidized and given loans, as some already are, to see them through. This would further push medicine into a socialistic mold, which may well be inevitable.

It may be inevitable for another reason: the financial crisis in the medical schools themselves. In 1970, of the 103 medical schools in the United States, more than half had received special federal grants to relieve financial distress. Among schools in financial difficulties were Johns Hopkins in Baltimore, George Washington and Georgetown in the District of Columbia, and St. Louis University. The reason is obvious. Tuition for medical students averaged $2,000 per year, while costs for the schools ran up to $16,000 per student per year. The actual cost of instruction for the students (excluding research programs and cost of delivering medical care to patients in the teaching hospitals) was about $5,000. It seems obvious that the government will eventually take over the financing of medical schools, and when that happens he who pays the piper will want to call the tune.

There are dangers in this course. In 1971, when the government of Quebec, Canada, had a row with medical specialists, it brought in a law that, in effect, conscripted physicians and forced them to practice under the Medicare law previously enacted. This had unexpected repercussions in education. As Dr. Bernard J. Perey, Professor of Surgery of Sherbrooke School of Medicine, put it, "this brutal attack" on liberties had caused physicians to lose all enthusiasm and desire to teach. "Vitally needed recruiting of new professors is deadlocked and teaching of medical students has begun to suffer," he claimed. "Professors will not have much difficulty in relocating themselves elsewhere."

This brings out a vital point often overlooked by politicians in handling the professions. You can make the doctor go to the clinic, but you cannot make him think. Also you cannot force students into medicine as you can into the army. If the profession becomes unattractive, it will be filled eventually by people of poor quality. Let Senator Kennedy and all similar socialized-medical fanatics take heed. Socialist Britain today exports British doctors to the United States. That supply will dry up if U.S. medicine becomes government-controlled.

2. The Circle Is Almost Complete

When I entered medical school in the early 1930s the general practitioner was in his heyday. But the storm of specialization was already a considerable cloud on the horizon. In North America in those days general practitioners were on the staffs of large hospitals, and, outside of a few stuffy medical schools, they did any procedure they felt qualified to tackle. Many took out appendices and repaired hernias. Others removed gallbladders for stones and did gastroenterostomies for peptic ulcers. One I know, who later became a world-famous surgeon, worked in an isolated area and even did some brain surgery. In addition, they delivered babies and treated medical problems which, in those days before antibiotics, were among the most unsatisfactory problems to handle.

After World War II the specialists took over, and with health plans coming into vogue, the patient could afford to go to them. Urbanization and the automobile altered the pattern of life. The lone GP was gradually replaced by clinics of GPs, with some of them getting specialty degrees while their partners kept the clinic going. The age of group practice was here.

The increasing cost of medical care and the depersonalization inevitable in mass-production techniques have made the consumer reconsider his attitudes. Most illnesses have a large psychological component. The patient needs a friend and the GP is becoming extinct. What to do? Bring the GP back after years of telling people that medical science had grown too big for any one man to understand? No, of course not! What was needed was a new kind of doctor—the family physician, certified as a specialist in primary care. The fact that primary care is essentially what the old GP used to do outside of operating in a hospital is nicely camouflaged by a lot of modern verbiage. This new guy is a specialist, you understand. He took several years of postgraduate training and he has a new degree. The new men seem to have forgotten that many GPs, myself included, took internships and some extra training in surgery and obstetrics in the old days and then often worked for an experienced man for a while before branching out. We did not have that paper on the wall, that's all.

The truth is that the circle is almost complete. The old father figure is spruced up in a new office with specialists at hand if he needs them. It may be more efficient as regards purely physical complaints, but I doubt if the psyche is as well handled as it used to be. For one thing, the doctor in a big-city practice nowadays probably knows little of the patient's background. People move around so much that, even with the best will in the world, it is not possible to know them.

What does this have to do with medical training? Just this: Some of the schools are shortening their courses and getting the students into contact with patients much earlier in their training. As Dr. Burgess of the new University of Missouri Medical School is reported by *American Medical News* to have said, "The goal of our school is to produce and graduate a different kind of physician who is an expert clinician but who is also aware of the psychological and social needs of the patients.''

That would be a good description of the GPs who taught me. Perhaps Dr. Burgess is too young to have known any.

3. The Long and the Short of It

In the time before I went to medical school in Toronto it took five years, after Grade 13, to graduate as a Bachelor of Medicine. Then a year and the Doctorate degree were added. For special students a B.A. in Biological and Medical Sciences was next, and I spent seven miserably long years acquiring the two degrees. After that came a rotating internship and then a residency in some specialty, at first three years, later four. So it was thirteen years from the end of high school (Grade 12, which is the U.S. termination) to the exalted pinnacle of a ''general'' specialist. Subspecialties took longer still. Had the trend continued, with the expansion of medical knowledge I could have predicted that the sub-sub-specialty diploma would arrive about the same time as the first heart attack. Fortunately, good sense, or fatigue, has prevailed and now everybody wants to shorten the length of both school and postschool study period.

Surprisingly, the computer era seems to have made this possible. The emphasis now is less on accumulation of facts in the head, which the computer remembers better, and more on how and where to acquire the necessary information and how to apply it logically. In other words, the emphasis is on learning to think medically.

Cutting the length of training can certainly be done. I have always felt that much of the college physics and chemistry and some of the detailed anatomy and physiology learned in the early years of medical school could have been eliminated. They could be enlarged upon in specialty years for those particular disciplines that require them. Dr. John Knowles in 1972 told the National Institute of Medicine in Washington, D.C., ''We have labored under the spell of science as a necessary and generally sole pre-condition in the educational process for a life in medicine. What is needed, instead, is broader undergraduate education that includes more of the humanities.''

I worked in Malawi with a British pathologist who had graduated from the University of Aberdeen, Scotland. He had been admitted to the medical course with a B.A. in English and no science. He learned the science that he required in medical school and is now a qualified specialist in the most scientific branch of medicine. I took a full course in humanities along with my science in pre-clinical studies and got a fine case of mental indigestion. I used very little of all that science as a GP. The humanities have been valuable to me personally and in enabling me to understand the viewpoints of those in other spheres of life. Otherwise I would have been nothing but a superior grade of technical officer.

There are some undesirable trends in this attempt to produce ''instant doctors.'' Some schools are allowing students to have many elective courses and several paths to the M.D. degree. In effect, this means that a young enthusiast determined to be a surgeon can start to specialize even before he graduates. To me this poses three questions:

1. Does he really know what he is best fitted to do at this early stage?

2. Will he be well rounded enough to recognize his limitations and that some problems lie outside his specialty?

3. If everyone does this, what happens to the distribution of doctors—will we have enough family physicians or will we have too many surgeons?

I remember very well that, like most youngsters, I wanted to be a surgeon. After six years of bloodshed in war I'd had enough of that and decided to do obstetrics. Then I ran out of money and had to do general practice. Finally, having tried a bit of everything, I became a pathologist. It would be harder for one who had specialized earlier to backtrack if he changed his mind.

The distribution of doctors of various types in our cities and rural areas will be a problem. Today, in our relatively free system, we already have serious maldistribution. Some years ago in Manitoba, Canada, the situation was so bad that it was proposed medical degrees should be withheld unless graduates did several years as GPs in remote or underserviced areas. The military services in the United States, chronically short of doctors, are asking for their own medical school to ensure a supply. It may be necessary in future to have a quota system—i.e., so many surgeons per state or city, so many family practitioners per 100,000 population. If that happens, we can expect to see frustrated would-be surgeons doing a poor job as country doctors. It might be better in the long run to educate more "all-purpose doctors" (I must give them a new title, of course), put them to work for several years after graduation and then pick out those with special abilities for further training. This is not a new idea. Some countries already insist that doctors do several years of general work before specializing. It will not be easy to arrange this, and it certainly will be unfair to some. It will delay specialization, but the doctors will probably be the better for it. It will, of course, be a form of regimentation and so socialization.

4. Overseas Education—the Great Training Robbery

Nowhere is the misdirection in medical training more evident than in the underdeveloped countries. Most of them have no medical schools of their own, and so they send off their bright sons and daughters to get an education, usually in Europe, North America or Australia. Where they go depends frequently on where they will be subsidized by the host country. So in recent years, with the politicians battling for friends in the strategic lands, students have gone to the most surprising places. For example, some from Kenya went to Russia and Bulgaria in spite of a severe language problem. Others went to Israel and India. A few ended in Germany or France or perhaps Scandinavia. The lucky ones went to the English-speaking countries and could start learning medicine right away. The confusion when they came back with different ideas and methods and different terminology played havoc with medical administration.

To the student the first result of going away was cultural shock. In fact, some students went on to "brain-fag syndrome," a condition described by several authors as "a psychosis or neurosis presumably precipitated by the stress of forcibly accelerated intellectual activity" and caused in part at least by the sudden transition from a peasant culture to a technological civilization much more competitive than what they had left.

Some years later those who had done well found themselves faced with going home. Now the shock was reversed. The pay in government service in their homeland was lower, the future was one of hard work in poor conditions for uncertain reward. Resentment in those who had stayed home against the newcomer with fancy ideas was liable to block promotion. Some never went home at all or got out again as soon as they could, which led to the second result. Some countries found that as many as half or more of their medically qualified natives stayed in or returned to the West. As an example, in 1969 about 900 Indian and Pakistani doctors emigrated to Great Britain. Many other foreign doctors went to the United States, where, if they met the immigration rules and passed the ECFMG (a qualifying test), they were welcomed to alleviate the "shortage" of interns and residents. The shortages in their own countries caused by the Western world's greed can be imagined.

Another result of overseas training is less obvious. Perhaps two examples will serve.

Some years ago in Africa a young, keen local doctor was sent away to England for advanced studies in internal medicine. On his return he dropped in to see me.

"Where will you be posted?" I asked.

He named a town up-country.

"You don't look too happy about it," I said.

"I expected it," he replied. "I only hope that they have some equipment I can work with. I'm not going to be a bush doctor."

He had forgotten that some of the finest medical work in his country had been done by men with little else but a stethoscope and their brains.

The second example is that of a young African who had had two years of training in anatomical pathology in Canada and then returned home for family reasons. Anxious to complete his studies, he scraped up the money to go back for the necessary two years in clinical pathology.

"Why go back to Canada? You can do it in other parts of Africa," I said.

"For one thing, the pay is good," he replied. In fact, he would make more in Canada as a trainee than I was getting as a specialist in his country.

"But the training is not really suitable," I protested. "In biochemistry and hematology this country can't afford auto-analyzers and automatic cell counters and all that fancy equipment. You will learn methods you will not be able to use here."

"Oh, we'll get equipment on a grant from the U.S.A., or the Russians might give us some for political reasons," he said airily. "In any case, I must have a degree that has some standing in the world."

From these examples it is obvious that many trainees returning home have strong personal ambitions and high expectations. Many who do come back go into private practice as soon as they can and make a lot of money. The government service and the rest of the country suffer. I find it hard to blame them when our own doctors do much the same.

To try to overcome these problems, governments with their own medical schools try to tailor their courses along lines more suited to the basic requirements of their population. However, in that regard there are difficulties, and I quote from an article by Dr. John Fry in the *Medical Tribune*, January 1971:

"There is a special problem in relation to the medical school and teaching hospitals in Africa. The hospital buildings are all modern and well built, often much too elaborate technically and architecturally for the country's needs. They usually are planned by European or American architects with little understanding of

Africa and they are usually much too large for their purpose.''

I can vouch for that. The problem is to convince ''Johnny-come-lately'' medical experts from the West that their ideas are far too grandiose and complicated. Even if they can be convinced, political egotism on the part of the leaders of the country demands only the best, and so the showplaces are built.

Countries that do not have enough professionals to staff these schools—and most do not—recruit doctors from the West to teach. In some ways this is good, but, for example, a professor who specializes in arteriosclerosis or lung cancer is like a duck out of water and has to learn what to talk about where he goes. Others insist on bringing expensive ideas with them and waste time and money before they wake up to the real situation. Some never do, as they are on short tours, on loan from some university, and don't have time to see the results of such policies. They leave, having done almost as much harm as good with their unrealistic teaching. Others spend more time on research in the fertile new fields than they do in teaching or treating patients. After all, the head of the department from which they came expects them to bring back some ''results'' of their time abroad.

A few stay longer but often find that young Western-trained native doctors are set above them in senior posts for reasons of prestige. Such men, lacking in experience and often grown anti-western from their years abroad, can make it difficult to keep things simple. They are quite sure they can handle anything the Westerner can and they ignore the obvious financial and technical problems which make this impractical.

The battle to train doctors in these countries is being lost for a quite unsuspected reason. Several years ago when Kenya set up a new medical school, it was calculated that the full output of doctors for the rest of this century would be absorbed by the fantastic increase in the population, so that the present ratio of one doctor to 30,000 people would not improve; in fact, it would deteriorate because of deaths of older doctors, emigration of younger ones and retirement of expatriates to their own lands. It would seem that medical care in the undeveloped lands can go only one way—backward.

5. Peer Review and the Tax-Free Travel Spree

After all the degrees have been earned and framed on the wall, learning is supposed to continue for the life of the doctor. For most doctors there is the stimulus of talking to associates in hospitals and clinics, but busy general practitioners may not have this privilege. Most read at least one medical periodical and consult their textbooks. A few ride along for years on what they learned in school plus what is gleaned from drug advertising. Partly because of such people and the rising discontent with medical services, malpractice suits are now common. In response, the American medical societies are talking about peer review, which means that all of us doctors are to be watched by our peers—i.e., other doctors—to be sure we are keeping up with the times and practicing good medicine.

It has been suggested by Dr. Gerald Dorman, formerly President of the American Medical Association, that our license to practice should lapse after a certain period and we should be reexamined before it is renewed. Dr. Dorman, being an old man, would not be involved much and so can make such a suggestion glibly. Having endured three years of residency training followed by a grueling examination at the age of forty-five for my pathology degree, I have personal knowledge of the sacrifice in time and mental anguish such a rule might extort, and I would flatly refuse to do it again. Most examinations test one's ability to remember reams of information one usually leaves in books to be read as necessary. They are not a true test of one's day-to-day ability to handle medical problems.

As far as I am concerned, submitting to such peer review is submitting to a type of Big Brotherism and an insult to my integrity. It is up to me to keep abreast and do good work. If I do not, I deserve to be sued, and probably will be. Furthermore, in our so-called democratic society I refuse to submit to such a review unless everybody else does. In other words, architects, engineers, plumbers, carpenters, lawyers and politicians should be peer-reviewed too. They can be just as dangerous to the public as doctors if they are incompetent. The results of peer-reviewing such people, especially the politicians, would be most enlightening.

Partly because of the peer-review mentality but mainly because all good ideas seem to grow and have to be improved upon by enthusiastic meddlers, we now have the disease I call conferencitis. Conferences of doctors, either general or special, are an old custom and have been useful as educational devices. However, I believe we are now having far too many and too elaborate meetings.

Originally these meetings were for the presentation of difficult or unusual cases or the reading of instructive papers, followed by discussion. This was, and still is, the procedure at the level of the local hospital or medical society. Then, with improved transportation, regional and national and international conferences became common. A newer idea, especially in such specialties as pathology, is to combine the traditional conference with workshops at which those interested can learn new techniques, operate new machines, test their diagnostic skill and so on.

The doctors' wives began to come along for a vacation and soon they were provided with museum visits, sight-seeing and shopping trips to pass the time. This led to a search for picturesque places in which to hold conferences or cheap package tours following the meeting. The latest gimmick I have heard about is the hiring of a cruise ship for a week or so of conferences, high living and touring. Of course, much of the cost is tax deductible, which encourages the physician to go, especially when airlines, tourist agencies and hotels fall over themselves to get the business.

Conferences of all kinds are prestige symbols now for the new nations. Millions are spent on new buildings that would have been better spent on patient care. Native doctors, newly appointed to high posts without the qualifications and experience that would have been required elsewhere, go off at frequent intervals to hob-nob with world authorities. They do not pay for it, of course. WHO does, or some other organization. It does not matter that the individual who goes is not competent or, for that matter, not particularly concerned with the subjects of the conference. The big thing is to be seen with the mighty and to sample the fleshpots of the world's great centers. The amount of money wasted in this way is appalling. I give one example.

From New Guinea a young native doctor was sent to Thailand for a conference on the treatment for protein deficiency in children. The cost was at least $800. A New Guinea native worker, making about $8.00 a week, will feed his family of several children on that. Thus the money spent on that conference would have kept his family for two years. In the hospital where the young doctor worked, there was a competent Australian pediatrician already handling numerous cases of the condition. It was not necessary to send the local man away at all. He could have learned all he needed to know from the Australian. As it happened, the whole trip was a waste to the country, for the young doctor left to go into another type of work shortly afterward.

In spite of all the nonsense, conferences are still basically useful training devices. Much can be learned from workshops and lectures, but there are now so many, on so many subjects, scheduled over three or four hectic days, that it is impossible to take in everything, even in narrow specialties. Furthermore, with notable exceptions, the presentation of papers, allotted ten minutes with supposedly five minutes more for discussion, makes a mockery of reasoned discourse. Usually one endures an unintelligible gabble by a poor speaker trying to cram an hour's talk into the time allotted. Inevitably he runs overtime and is buzzed off the podium like a contestant in an old-fashioned amateur hour. Far more could be gained by reading the same paper in the quiet of a library back home.

My old professor of pathology once said to me, "Sam, I go to conferences to meet people and talk to them over a drink in the hotel room. Most of the papers are worthless." This may be too harsh a judgment, but it calls into question the worth of the whole frantic procedure as a postgraduate educational device. It can certainly do without all the hoopla and get back to a simpler format. But how many would attend in that case?

7

The Replacement Racket

1. The Greatest Show on Earth

EVERY DAY IN THE UNITED STATES 1,500 people die of heart attacks. Five hundred more die of strokes. Hundreds of thousands survive the first attack and live in fear, waiting for the dreadful pain to strike again. The fortunate die fast. Others gasp their way to death as their damaged hearts pound between their tortured lungs.

The stroke victim, partly paralyzed, totters about with drooling mouth and vacant stare, perhaps incontinent and unable to communicate properly, a nuisance to himself and to everyone around him.

The basic cause of both these diseases is arteriosclerosis, in my opinion almost 100 percent preventable (see Chapter 12). But how have our experts approached the problem? The biochemists have tried to find the cause by delving into the abstruse complexities of fat and sugar metabolism, only to get lost in a maze of enzymes. The physiologists worry about blood pressure and fluid balances. The surgeons, forthright souls that they are, have come up with a really dramatic attack. New Hearts for old, they cry! For damaged brains there is no such answer, of course.

In December 1967 Dr. Christiaan Barnard, in Capetown, South Africa, did the first heart transplant on a Mr. Washkansky, who lived about two weeks. Barnard followed soon afterward with the world's second transplant, on Phillip Blaiberg, an Afrikaner dentist. Barnard's *tour de force* created headlines around the world and a rush to repeat his success in a dozen centers. By September 1971 a total of 167 transplants had been recorded, but only 22 patients were still alive. The longest survival at that time was thirty months.

Was it worthwhile? Dr. Blaiberg lived for nineteen months and, according to his twenty-two-year-old daughter, his life was "a hell," his wife suffered "more than any other woman I know" and her own life was "messed up." Part of this was undoubtedly due to the publicity.

Of the 22 survivors, 9 were able to return to work—i.e., about 5 percent of all cases went back to a useful life: a poor return for the tremendous investment in medical skill, time and money. The fatalities were due to graft rejection and infection, with rejection the main cause of death in those who lived longest. This is important for two reasons. It means that the body continues trying to get rid of the new heart, and that drug suppression of the immune reaction must continue indefinitely.

It will be argued that this problem can be overcome. Dr. Stinson of the Stanford Medical Center in California now claims a 30 percent survival rate at two years after operation. His cases are carefully selected, of course. Let us look at the logistics of the problem.

2. Cheap at Any Price?

When Barnard was in his glory it was estimated that a heart transplant cost $30,000. If the patient survived, it cost thousands more to continue immunosuppression and to bring the patient back for frequent reexamination. For a rich man this may be worthwhile, but what about others? Should families be pauperized and Medicare plans be bankrupted to keep alive a lot of cripples? And what of the medical manpower problem? It takes two surgical teams for a transplant, one to remove the donor's heart and the other to put it into the recipient. It takes twenty-four-hour observation by medical specialists, nurses, laboratory technicians and others until the crisis is over. It requires the use of a fantastically complicated Intensive Care Unit at charges up to $500 per day (the doctor's bill is separate).

Even if all these difficulties are overcome, the major problem remains. Where do we get all the new hearts? Let us suppose we could save 10 percent of all the daily deaths from heart attack by transplants. We would need more than 50,000 a year. If we could, by some miracle, extract the hearts of all the motor-traffic victims and store them, we would still not have enough, because many of them, too, have diseased hearts.

One suggestion is to use the hearts of animals such as the pig. The problems of immunosuppression are unsolved as I write, but it could happen. When that day comes, and assuming that two surgeons working as a team can do five transplants a day (1,000 a year) before they drop with fatigue, it will require 100 cardiac surgeons doing nothing else for five days a week, an assembly-line torture that only a sadist could devise, to save 50,000 middle-aged crocks each year (if they all survive!). The other 500,000 will still die.

Knowing this, and believing as I do that the whole business is preventable, I can only agree with Dr. John R. Miles, who wrote in the *Medical Tribune* on March 30, 1971, that in prevention lies true progress and that "viewed in this light, organ transplantation might be described as the most brilliant surgical irrelevance of the century."

Fortunately, new methods of surgery of the coronary arteries, the vessels of the heart itself, are showing promising results and this may serve until prevention of arteriosclerosis relegates all these procedures to the medical museum.

3. Old Wine in New Bottles

In the other organ systems the picture is equally gloomy. Of 136 liver transplants done since 1963, only 12 were alive in September 1971. The longest-lived survivor had lasted twenty-nine months. Of 23 pancreas transplants for severe diabetes of children, none had survived. In kidney disease the picture is better. *Newsweek*, in an article on December 20, 1971, reported that the success rate for transplants from live donors was 70 percent and for cadaver kidneys was 50 percent. The cost of treatment was about \$25,000 per case as opposed to a kidney-dialysis cost of \$200 per treatment or \$25,000 annually. Here too we run into the problem of where to get suitable kidneys. The supply is far smaller than the demand, and patients wait for months until one can be found.

The problem of whom to select for a kidney transplant, since the supply is insufficient, raises ethical, legal and political problems. This is one place where, like it or not, someone has to "play God." Good health (other than the kidney disease) plus a sound mental and psychological constitution are necessary if the transplant is to be worth while. The decision as to whether or not one patient would be of more benefit to society than another is carefully skirted in most of the discussions I have read. We, in our democratic society, are most reluctant to state that one citizen is worth more than another unless, of course, one is a national hero or a "great man." Transplantation is a highly unsatisfactory solution for these reasons, and the sooner a mechanical device can be built (in the absence of prophylaxis or cure), the better.

As I write, it is reported that a plastic capsule containing an absorbent material may be used instead of dialysis and could possibly do away with the need for transplants. Until prevention of kidney infection reaches a satisfactory level, this sort of procedure may be the answer.

To date, in all major organs except the kidneys, transplantation has a very poor record of success at an unbearably high cost in money, medical manpower and mental and physical anguish.

When we consider that the same effort and money, expended in investigation and preventive treatment, might have come up with a cure to some of the diseases, then we have to view transplant surgery as inferior therapy. The disease that caused the original organ to deteriorate may still be present in the patient's tissues and blood, as in the case of arteriosclerosis, and affect the new one. Putting old wine into new bottles may fool the customer, but only for a while.

8

The Customer Is Always Right

1. Do Something, Doctor!

DOCTORS ARE PEOPLE who have to make a living. Like everyone else, they try to be successful at it. In socialist countries or in salaried positions elsewhere the pressure may be less. In fact, in such situations the physician is often motivated to keep people out of his office because he knows they are not sick and they give him more work with no more pay. Still he cannot risk too many complaints, and so even in these situations the customer is usually right.

The honest doctor, and I firmly believe most are honest, does his best to ensure that patients are helped, and never hurt, by what he does, but sometimes the thinking is misdirected. Much depends on the type of practice and the nature of the patients he treats. When in general practice I found, as all doctors do, that a patient wanted me to "do something" for him—something better than "just advice." He had to have a prescription or an injection or a "treatment." The problem was to ensure that if he could not be helped, he at least would not be harmed. This is where the line may be crossed—where, I feel, medicine goes wrong.

2. Silicones and Sex

In recent years we have gone from the era of the uplift brassiere, with its hint of hidden delights, to topless waitresses. Topless they are not. In fact, I will never forget the remark attributed to a famous movie producer as he gazed into the bosom of an equally famous star: "My God, they forgot to milk her!"

Now, a few lucky women are big and shapely in the bosom, but anyone who has lived in New Guinea, or Africa in the old days, realizes that the mammary glands come in many shapes and sizes and most of them are not attractive. In fact, in such areas breasts are useful objects and are not considered sexual adornments.

In the West, unfortunately, the breast is highly sexual and, with clothes gradually vanishing, at least on the beaches, it is important that it be beautiful. In the old days a clever plastic surgeon could do a lot with his knife and skilled stitching. Nowadays we have silicones in various forms.

If silicones were completely inert, one might feel no twinge of conscience as skillfully inserted pads or other prostheses converted a physically and mentally depressed young woman into a pouter pigeon. But they are not all inert, and there are numerous case histories of dreadful abscesses and disfiguring scars resulting from such operations. Furthermore, nobody can say what the result of thirty or forty years of carrying these implants around will be. Can we be absolutely certain that they are not carcinogenic or that their presence will not stimulate a latent carcinoma?

Perhaps I am old-fashioned, but I question the ethics of surgical procedures utilizing foreign body insertion where the end result is merely to gratify an ego or enable an entertainer to get a job. A simple mammoplasty or a face lift or nose straightening may deceive others as to the patient's true physical characteristics, but such deception is part of our lives. Corsets, wigs, brassieres and so on are acceptable deceptions. We learn to look behind them. They do not usually hurt the wearer. We cannot yet be certain that foreign-body insertions will not.

3. Fibber McGee's Closet

Older North Americans will remember the famous comedy team of Fibber McGee and Molly, who worked for years on radio, in movies and eventually on television. Fibber used to dispose of unwanted articles in a closet so full that he had to close the door with great care. Invariably, during the program he would get excited, rush to the closet to get something, fling open the door and vanish in a cascade of bric-a-brac. The scene always excited a great wave of laughter. Unfortunately, the cupboard I want to open is crowded too, but is no laughing matter.

Over the years since World War II medical scientists have discovered dozens of analgesics, antibiotics, antihistamines, antidepressants, anti-anything you can think of except an anti-anti. As the drug-company literature and the news media reported each great new discovery, so the patient expected and often demanded that the doctor prescribe it for him. Some of these wonder drugs could be bought without prescription at the drug store. After each illness there would probably be a few capsules left over, and so when little Willie got sick, his mother or a neighbor would say, "Oh, my husband had exactly the same complaint last June and this new medicine fixed him up." Willie got the capsules left over. He probably got better because most illnesses are self-limited and so one more person was sensitized to one more drug, or one more bacterium became resistant to it.

The story is a simplification, but the problem is serious. In the early days of these drugs, especially the antibiotics, professors of bacteriology and medicine used to say, "You must isolate the organism and do sensitivity tests, then use the antibiotic to which it is sensitive." This is a counsel of perfection, as any general practitioner knows. One cannot leave a sick child with a sore throat or incipient pneumonia lying in bed for forty-eight hours while a throat swab is being processed, first to grow the bacteria and then to determine their sensitivity. So short cuts are taken. The best way is to look at a slide made from the swab. Often the organism is recognizable, and if, for example, it turns out to be pneumococcus, one can give penicillin at once, since pneumococci are sensitive to that antibiotic. However, this may not be possible, and so, while waiting for the laboratory results, the doctor will prescribe an antibiotic that, from experience, he hopes will work.

When Mother does the prescribing and then calls in the doctor a day or so later, the problem is more difficult. Her treatment may suppress but not kill the bacteria. They will not grow on the blood agar plates in the laboratory, but they can still grow inside the patient. The doctor then has to work partially in the dark. We see this sort of thing all too often among white people in the tropics. I remember one man who felt feverish. He took a couple of antimalarial tablets, but was not greatly improved. The next day he came to the hospital. The blood smear did not show any malarial parasites and the doctor spent precious days trying to discover what was wrong. The man was now seriously ill. At last, four days later, the parasites reappeared in the blood in their millions and a technician, looking for something else, spotted them and reported the fact. Antimalarial treatment in proper dosage was given and the patient survived, but it was a near thing.

We are now into a new era, the era of iatrogenic disease, which means disease caused by doctors. But the patient must be considered an accessory to the crime. We do not know the sites of action of some of the drugs we now use. We are finding out that some are synergistic—i.e., the effect of two or more drugs prescribed at the same time may be greater than the sum of the effects separately or, worse still, the combination may result in some quite unexpected effect. For instance, there are some well-known agents called mono-amine oxidase inhibitors which are used to combat severe psychological depression. If while under treatment the patient eats certain foods such as cheese or wine which contain so-called pressor amines, the result may be a great rise in blood pressure which could be fatal in a patient already suffering from hypertension. There are many other possible combinations with unfortunate results—for example, the combination of alcohol with some tranquillizers. When we remember that today the average American patient in a hospital receives as many as fifteen or twenty different medications and takes some home too, we should not be surprised if once in a while the contents of that medical closet bury him.

To my mind, there should be no "leftovers" in the medicine chest to use up. The man who can devise a pill that will crumble away a week after the patient is cured will have the blessing of every doctor alive. The drug companies will love him too.

4. The Annual Exam and Eisenhower

Some years ago there was a great surge of enthusiasm for annual medical examinations. It has not quite died out, but we are fortunate in that either sense or inertia is beginning to prevail. If we consider that perhaps half the 400,000 or so doctors in America could be used to question and examine the more than 200 million people, then each doctor would do 1,000 people per year. A thorough check-up, including ordering and considering basic laboratory tests, chest X-ray and so on, would certainly take a half-hour. Thus each doctor would spend 500 hours yearly in physical examinations alone, or ten weeks at the doctor's usual working pace of fifty-to-sixty-hour weeks. And for what?

He would find an occasional lump in a breast that a woman had not noticed, or a suspicious cervical smear. He would certainly note arteriosclerosis and emphysema, but since over 50 percent of Americans die of the results of arteriosclerosis and most older people have it, the finding is not noteworthy. He might pick up a lung cancer, but early detection has not so far lowered the death rate dramatically; stopping smoking and clearing the air are much more effective. He will not find stomach or intestinal cancer, as the ordinary annual examination cannot afford to include such investigations.

Let me tell you a bit of history, because I happened to be there. In 1954-55 I was a resident in pathology at Fitzsimons Army Hospital in Denver, Colorado. Mrs. Eisenhower's mother lived in Denver and so the President came to visit and he also came to Fitzsimons for his annual physical examination, with experts flown in from as far away as Washington, D.C. The examination was much more complete than most people get and included plenty of laboratory tests for us to do. At the end President Eisenhower was pronounced to be fit, in very good condition for a man of his age. About ten days later he had the first of a series of massive heart attacks and strokes that eventually killed him. So much for the worth of the annual physical examination in prognosis, at least as far as arteriosclerosis is concerned.

I thought when I wrote this I might be alone in my opinion, but in January 1972 Dr. John G. Smillie, Assistant Director of Kaiser Permanente operations in Northern California, stated that "an annual physical is sort of like motherhood and cleanliness but no one knows for sure what it does." He based his opinions on consultations with doctors in his organization who were involved in such examinations. He made other comments, among them: "You should have an initial complete examination. As long as you enjoy robust positive health it is not necessary to have an annual check-up." And another: "The most effective ways of staying healthy longer involve sensible living habits."

Another boom in recent years has been in cytology, which has now become a science of its own with its faithful disciples. Cervical cytology, of course, should be included in the physical examination and, for the same reasons as the annual examination, is of limited benefit. Some women have been saved from death by recognition of early cancer. Others with suspicious smears have gone on for years if the gynecologist has been strong-willed enough to wait before operating. Some have had the suspicious findings return to normal.

There is good statistical evidence that cancer of the cervix was on the decline before all this furor over cervical smears, so that the cytologists cannot take all the credit for the reduction in cases. It has something to do with early age of beginning sexual intercourse, number of partners and hygiene. Perhaps the disease is viral, contracted years before the cancer becomes visible. In such case it seems likely to increase with the new sexual permissiveness, as venereal disease has done, and the matter should be a public health problem rather than a curative medical one. However, until a vaccine is discovered, we will have millions of women getting millions of smears and taking up doctors' time that would be better spent elsewhere.

5. Much Ado About Little

In the Western world, where the major health problems are insoluble until we change our way of life (see Chapter 12), we have accepted these diseases with minimal fuss compared to the hell we would raise if, for example, the same number of deaths were due to cholera. Having done this, we can get excited about diseases which, to put it bluntly, are so rare we should get on with something more important. I refer to the genetic metabolic diseases such as phenylketonuria, with an incidence of one in 25,000 births, and cystic fibrosis, which is more common but still rare. Part of the interest lies in the recent advances in biochemistry and genetics which have enabled us to do intricate investigations and devise reasonably simple tests for their detection. Nevertheless, the fuss over them is out of all proportion to their importance. This is not so in some other inherited conditions, such as sickle-cell anemia, which came to America with the slaves and is an important cause of anemia. Similarly, thalassemia is not too uncommon in Mediterranean peoples and porphyria among the numerous Afrikaans descendants of the original Dutch settlers who included carriers of the disease in their small company.

The problem with these conditions is propagation and perpetuation. The sickle-cell trait had survival value in malarious countries, since the parasites did not thrive in the abnormal blood. It has no such value in America, and those who have the full-blown disease, as opposed to the trait, are chronically ill and a burden to everyone. A tedious but brilliant series of biochemical investigations recently completed by Dr. Makio Murayama of the National Institute of Health has explained the nature of the abnormal hemoglobin molecule and, based on this, a way to reverse or prevent the sickling (i.e., collapse) of the red cells. Now it seems that sicklers can live to grow up and beget more with the same defect. In a world already overcrowded this seems a dubious accomplishment, but I have no doubt that the parents will demand that their children be kept alive along with all the other genetic misfits. This is one place where compulsory sterilization might be considered, but the customer will never allow it, at least not yet.

6. Choose the Sex, It's Your Child

The problem mentioned above may be solved as an unexpected bonus from our consumers' demands. It is already possible to tell if a child in the womb is of the same blood group as the mother, and it was a very short step for the cytologist to tell if it would be a normal male or female. The new permissiveness and ease of doing abortions lead us to the next step. If we do not like the sex of the fetus, then we discard it. Later on we will probably be able, by pretreatment, to determine the sex we want at the time of conception or shortly thereafter. Since some of the genetic diseases are sex-linked, it will be possible to prevent the birth of a child who can transmit the defect.

Picking the sex of your child could result in a serious imbalance of one sex or the other—for example, in countries such as India where fathers want sons to perform the last rites for them. It might help the overpopulation problem, but would undoubtedly require rethinking of our moral standards.

To sum up: The demands of the consumer have a much greater influence on the quality, quantity and direction of medical practice than most people will admit. Some demands are reasonable. Others are foolish or frivolous. Some are downright harmful. It will require discipline on the part of both doctors and consumers to ameliorate the situation. Are we capable of it?

9

Anything Free Is Expensive

1. The High Cost of Comfort

AS WE KNOW, medical care in hospitals is appallingly expensive these days. Many politicians attempt to put the blame on doctors and point to high fees, utilization of hospitals when outpatient care would do, excessive ordering of procedures, tests and drugs and so on. Some of this is true, but on the question of overly high doctors' fees in the United States, a bit of perspective helps.

Senator Abraham Ribicoff in an article in the *Saturday Review*, August 22, 1970, stated, "Doctors' fees during the 1960's rose twice as fast as the general cost of living. . . ." This is a typical politician's ploy to put doctors in a bad light. To the layman it sounds like sheer greed on their part. However, in the same publication a year later Harry Schwartz of the *New York Times* said, "Between 1967 and 1970 the consumer price index shows that physicians' fees rose an average of 21.4 percent or *almost exact-*

ly the same percentage by which average hourly earnings of workers on private non-agricultural payrolls increased over the same period." [Italics mine.] So if the doctor is overcharging, everyone else is too except the farm worker and the government employee.

Ribicoff admitted that, compared with the cost five years previously, 18 percent of the increase in the nation's health bill was due to increased population and 47 percent to inflation, technology, wage increases for hospital employees and just plain higher charges. He admitted that *35 percent came from more services provided per person*. The latter statement is the real shocker. I seriously doubt if the morbidity and mortality figures today, as compared with five years ago, can justify a 35 percent increase in costs. In other words, the money may have made illness pleasanter but very little safer. Can we afford it?

2. Die Quick or Live in Penury

Catastrophic-care insurance is much in the news, and certainly something of that nature must be provided to everyone if possible. No ordinary family can bear the costs of prolonged illness these days. Even ten years ago a disabling heart attack, stroke or accident, where the unfortunate victim dragged on for weeks, was a financial as well as an emotional disaster. I remember one case involving a relative of mine. The husband, a retired minister, suffered a stroke. He was unconscious, requiring twenty-four-hour nursing service that was costing $100 per day. His pension was $150 per month. The surgeons operated, hoping to save his life. They succeeded, but he remained unconscious, a vegetable, for another six months before he died. Fortunately, the family doctor found out that he had had just enough service in the Army in World War I to qualify as a veteran. He was transferred at once to a Veterans Administration hospital, saving the widow from a hospital bill that could have been as much as $18,000, the equivalent of ten years' total pension. This case had a happier ending than many others. It illustrates the need for catastrophe insurance, but it also illustrates something people do not usually consider: someone else paid that hospital bill—i.e., the taxpayer. It was free to the family, expensive to the country.

3. Money for Jam

One of the solutions to the high cost of medical care is group insurance. We all know about Blue Cross and recently a great deal of attention has been focused on the Kaiser Permanente health plan, which has a somewhat different basis. In Canada some twenty-five years ago health-insurance plans were started, under the control of the doctors in various provinces, and the one in British Columbia got going just as I left the army in 1946 and, needing money badly, went into general practice. The idea sounded good. Each employee of a firm paid a monthly medical fee for himself and his family. The firm put up a similar amount. Patients went to doctors in the usual way, but the doctor billed the insurance plan.

The first few months in this tiny isolated company town I made about $500 per month, mostly in industrial-accident fees and a company retainer. Then the plan came in. The next month I made $1,000 and it never dropped back again. To me, in those days, it was a fortune. My office was full of people, but I noticed that very few were really sick. They wanted to talk to me and be reassured, or they wanted to save a few pennies by getting "free medicine" instead of buying something in the drug store. Others went off to the big city to see specialists they could not previously have afforded. In a couple of years every woman with uterine fibroids had had them removed; tonsils and adenoids had been discarded; old hernias had been fixed. It was a great time for the people, but the plan almost went broke and would have without stringent new rules, brought in after I had left in disgust to do some real medicine at a much lower salary.

4. The Army Knows All About It

All this could have been predicted. We knew about it in the Army during World War II. In 1939 I was assigned to a Royal Canadian Air Force Manning Depot where the eager young volunteers first came. Faced with drills, regimentation, KP and no airplanes, they were disgusted. But we had to keep them there long enough to make soldiers out of the undisciplined mob. Alone in the hospital, I had wards full of genuinely ill airmen, but the sick parade each morning was a different matter. On Mondays, tired after weekend leave, hung over or trying to avoid the weekly route march, 120 "sick" men waited outside my office. On Fridays, since those on sick parade lost weekend passes, I might see 20. On Sunday, when the men could sleep in, it might be less than 10. Sick parade, costing nothing, was used as it is today in places that have medical plans or socialized medicine, to further interests that have little to do with organic illness.

5. The Three-Minute Miracle Men

In socialized countries such as Great Britain and Sweden the patient pays very little in direct charges for medical care. Thus he is not deterred from making frequent visits for trivial complaints. Doctors' offices are so crowded with patients in some cities that if visits were counted and divided into the hours worked, the time allotted per patient would be three or four minutes. It does not work out that way, of course, since renewal of a prescription or signing an off-work slip takes less time and a sick man gets more. Nevertheless, to get through the day, the harried doctor hurries along like an assembly-line mechanic. There is no time to soothe the worried or frightened, no time for the intensive questioning or deliberation that may uncover the basic cause of some illness. As in the assembly line, if the patient is an "unusual model," he must be put aside to be worked on later or, more likely, referred to the presumably less harried specialist.

This scenario is carried to the point of lunacy in the underdeveloped countries whose politicians point proudly to their "free medical care." In Malawi, formerly Nyasaland, before independence there was a small charge for outpatient visits. The outpatient clinic in the country's largest hospital was remodeled shortly before the great day to handle 300 patients daily, which at that time was more than adequate. With typical demagoguery, free medical care was brought in by the new regime. Today, some eight years later, the clinic processes at least 1,500 and frequently over 2,000 people daily with approximately the same staff of medical assistants, nurses and doctors and a budget for supplies and medicines little larger than before independence. The quality of the medical care can be imagined.

The situation is equally bad as regards inpatients. In the same hospital in May 1971 in a surgical ward with 58 beds there were 110 patients; 52 were lying on the floor. Proper nursing care and hygiene were impossible. Many inpatients were terminal or chronic cases with nowhere to go except back to their huts. There was no money for extra beds in the hospital and none for the extra food to take care of the overflow. The politicians didn't care. The people had been given free treatment. The rest was up to the medical staff.

The sad part is that the people themselves must take much of the blame for this dreadful overcrowding. Most of those who stand for half a day waiting to be seen are not really sick by African standards. By this I mean that since everyone has worms of some kind, spleens enlarged and tender from chronic malaria, and energy sapped by poor nutrition or anemia, they are problems for the preventive medical teams and not for the hospital staff. It is noticeable that the crowd at the clinic is halved in inclement weather. Really ill people would still come, I am sure. Dr. John Fry, in the *Medical Tribune* of January 1971, stated in regard to East Africa, "Most of those attending [clinics] are suffering from surprisingly minor ailments, much more trivial than those seen in general practice in Great Britain, such as minor cuts and bruises, colds, coughs and sore throats and diarrhoea." As regards the work of the medical assistants who staff these clinics, he says, "The speed of their work is impressive but less so when one realises that very few examinations are made and almost no tests are carried out. 'Spot Diagnosis' based on a quick history is the basis of their work." This confirms my own observations in Africa and elsewhere. It points out the fallacy of substituting free care for payment of some kind, and the other fallacy that medical assistants can be used instead of doctors to provide adequate service. They can be used, but only under direct control.

In the same way, in the West those who crowd into the doctor's office with symptoms of arteriosclerosis, lung disease and many other conditions are also basically public health problems, as we will see in Chapter 12.

6. Quality or Quantity? We Cannot Have Both

In America, in group medical schemes, the situation is not much better. In April 1970, in an article in *Scientific American*, Dr. Sidney Garfield of the Kaiser Permanente group wrote, in part, "Only after years of experience did we discover that *the elimination of the fee is practically as much of a barrier to early sick care as the fee itself*. The reason is that when we removed the fee we removed the regulator of flow into the system and put nothing in its place. The result is an uncontrolled flow of well, worried-well, early sick, and sick people into our point of entry—the doctor's appointment—on a first come first served basis that has little relation to a priority of need. The impact of this demand overloads the system and, *since the well and the worried-well people are a considerable proportion of our entry mix, the usurping of available doctor's time by the healthy people actually interferes with the care of the sick*." [Italics mine.] I could have told him that thirty years earlier, but I didn't have a computer to prove it statistically.

As I mention elsewhere, Dr. Garfield and others are trying to get around this problem by screening patients, putting them through machine-processed questionnaires, batteries of biochemical and other analyses and interviews with physician's assistants. If patients pass these hurdles, they can see the doctor. This is hardly the kind of friendly, intimate medical attention most people hope to get. It is what they deserve for abusing the system.

7. It's Papa Who Pays

In 1971, the first year that all Canadian provinces were enrolled in the Medicare program, it was estimated that the federal government would pay out $550 million. The provinces would equal that amount. This is about $50 per year for every Canadian.

In 1970 Medicaid in the United States paid out $5,200 million in medical services to 15 million poor people whose needs might otherwise not have been met, according to the director of the Medical Services Administration. This is roughly $350 per person and, being poor, they probably did not pay taxes. Most of the states were struggling with severe financial crises in their Medicaid programs. Of 34 states contacted by *American Medical News* in January 1971, 24 were running deficits and only 5 expected to expand welfare and Medicaid programs.

The experience of the European countries with socialistic medical programs is much the same. All programs have cost far more than was originally expected. For example, in Sweden health expenditures increased between 1950 and 1966 by 614 percent while those in the United States rose by 174 percent. I do not propose to get into the argument of fee-for-service versus governmental control of medicine. I have worked as a salaried employee of various governmental agencies since I left private practice in 1949. I will say this: Unless the patient is made to realize the costs of medical care—and the obvious way is to require him pay enough in direct fees to make him think—then medical care will be abused and will be expensive to the taxpayer. In poor countries I have heard it said that the people cannot afford to pay. Somehow they find money or goods for the witch doctor who will not see them without payment in advance. If they do not have cash, let them provide goods or services such as a blood donation or work on community projects. Free medical care is also expensive in terms of wrong diagnoses, inadequate treatments and harassment of emotions in the assembly-line clinics and packed hospitals. It is time for some discipline and a lot less political haymaking about the "inherent right of all people to medical care." If inherent right means "existing in someone as a natural and inseparable quality" (Webster's Dictionary), then human beings have only one inherent medical right—the right to die.

10

The Love-Hate Relationship

1. The Dedication Concept

EVERYWHERE I GO, sooner or later I read about or hear somebody sniping at doctors. A fight has been going on in Australia between "representatives of the people," which usually means politicians anxious for publicity or labor leaders green with envy, and the general practitioners, who are insisting on raising their fees, as everybody else is doing these days.

Later I will discuss this question of filthy-rich doctors, but here I want to refer to the peculiar idea in most people's minds that doctors are "dedicated." In the ordinary dictionary meaning of "devoted to some special work" this is quite true, but to many people it has semi-religious connotations, as if we were members of some monastic order, which, by derivation, is taken to mean we are above mundane considerations such as a decent standard of living, reasonable hours of work, education for our kids, money for retirement and so on. We are not. We are, as a group, as honest as or perhaps more honest than most, we work far harder than most people, but, aside from missionaries, we do not have some divine call.

In the old days the doctor, like the minister, was on a special plane of society and treated with reverence and respect. With increasing education and sophistication of ordinary people, this respect was eroded until today there is a curious love-hate relationship between doctors and the public. When I came out of World War II and went into general practice I ran into this situation. There was one particular patient who had made frequent calls to my partner but never paid his bills. He was warned, when the last call was made, that he was well and therefore no longer our responsibility and that we did not want him as a patient. Shortly thereafter he walked in on an open day and demanded to see the doctor. The nurse brought him to me, as being more hard-hearted than my kindly senior partner. I asked a few questions to make sure this was not an emergency and then I said, "I'm sorry, we cannot take you as our patient."

"I've been Dr. P——'s patient for years," he said angrily. "Why can't you see me?"

"You never pay your bills. This is not an emergency. I refuse to handle your case."

"But you have to," he spluttered. "You swore an oath of Hippo . . . Hippo . . . something. You can't refuse."

"I can, and do," I said. "Now please excuse me, I'm busy."

Both legally and ethically I was within my rights. I risked having my name blackened in the community by his outraged complaints. But we are not saints. We need to live, and after all the expense and years of education, we feel entitled to live as well as less qualified businessmen, engineers, lawyers and, yes, plumbers and carpenters. The sooner the public accepts this and forgets the dedication concept, the better our relationship will be.

I might say here I have worked for years in the tropics for salaries and in conditions very few American tradesmen would accept. I say it only to show that in this section I am not defending my own position but that of my fellow doctors.

2. I'll Call My Lawyer

One consequence of the souring of relationships between doctors and laymen is the malpractice suit. It is almost unknown in developing countries, is uncommon but increasing in Britain and the former Dominions and has almost disrupted normal relationships in parts of the United States such as California, where several years ago it was reported that each year one doctor in four was sued. Regardless of the cause, the result of this has been a rocketing of medical malpractice insurance into the stratosphere of high finance. The costs, as in all business, are eventually passed on to the consumer, so Mr. John Doe pays more for medical attention in the end.

The situation became so bad that in the last year or two some insurance companies were refusing to reinsure physicians in high-risk categories such as anesthetists and certain categories of surgeon. Who could blame them when juries, with the firm conviction that doctors should not make so much money, were awarding million-dollar convictions? In Hawaii in 1970 about 250 of the approximately 1,000 physicians were refused insurance. It was bad too in New Mexico, so bad that it was estimated 20 young doctors did not enter the state to practice because they could not get liability coverage.

In self-defense the doctors set up a group-insurance program sponsored and watched by the state medical association in conjunction with a major insurance carrier which agreed to take the risk provided 85 percent of the doctors in the state had joined up by the end of four years. Rates varied for different specialties—e.g., in New Mexico a doctor doing surgery paid $651 per year for coverage, but a plastic surgeon had to spend $3,950 per year.

Another way of counterattacking was the countersuit or threat of action by lawyers hired by medical associations or groups. This frightened off some people who were making a racket out of malpractice suits alleging improper advances by the doctor to a female patient, improper prescribing resulting in mental or physical distress, indecent interference with a patient under anesthesia and so on.

3. Tests I Never Look At

There is a new kind of medicine being practiced nowadays in sophisticated countries. It has been called "defensive medicine" and is an anathema to all decent doctors as well as to patients. I put the blame for this terrible misdirection in medicine largely on the general public, but the doctors cannot escape some group responsibility.

In Chapter 12 I quote figures from studies several groups of medical specialists made of the competence of general practitioners. Far too many failed to pass the standards set as necessary for proper practice. Doctors such as these are asking for malpractice suits and here the public has a legitimate grievance. To overcome this, medical associations have put forward ideas such as relicensing examinations, peer reviews, compulsory attendance at seminars and so on. Meanwhile the battle between the doctor and the patient goes on.

There are numerous manifestations of defensive medicine. When I was a country doctor I used to see female patients alone, examine them in various stages of undress alone, administer medications to intimate areas and so on. The company I worked for would not hire a nurse and I could not afford one. I would flatly refuse to do that today.

My introduction to defensive medicine came in 1946 in the same practice. I saw and treated a man who had sprained his ankle in the mill. He recovered quickly and I sent my bill to the Workmen's Compensation Board.

The medical administrator rang me up. "You haven't submitted your bill for X-ray," he said, knowing that I had a small machine provided by the company.

"I didn't take one. It was a simple sprain."

"You should have," he replied.

"Look, you asked me to keep costs down," I protested.

"I did, but who knows whether or not this man will come back years from now and claim he has a chronic synovitis dating from an undetected fracture—something he probably got out hunting or playing ball—which he blames on this injury?"

"My God, man, if that's the case, I'll have to X-ray all sprains."

"You will, and we will gladly pay for it. You must be able to prove to a jury, by showing them an X-ray, that there was no fracture. They won't necessarily take your opinion. They will believe the X-ray."

Not long ago a friend of mine, a New York surgeon, took a year off to work for a mission in Malawi. He sent in a request for a battery of laboratory tests and when I rang him up to ask if he needed them he laughed.

"Sorry, Sam, I forgot I wasn't at home."

"Yeah, I know. We haven't got an autoanalyzer here. But what do you want all those tests for?"

"I don't really. Back home I order tests I never look at."

"For God's sake, why do you do that?"

"Look, Sam, a surgeon is fair game back home. If something goes wrong and the patient sues me, I have to prove I did everything possible to ensure his safety. Lawyers make a lot out of figures, and people have a lot more faith in lab tests than you or I have."

"I'm afraid that's true. But out here it isn't necessary."

I leave you to look at your last hospital bill and remember that, as a member of the public, you brought a lot of the cost on yourself.

4. He's Making a Fortune

It is generally agreed, except by the medical profession, that doctors are rich and greedy and charge too much. Some of us are guilty. Most are not. With the advent of Medicare in the United States there was a terrible outcry when it was found that a few doctors made well over $100,000 yearly from it. The fact that some of these men worked literally day and night was ignored. The biggest "offender" turned his books over to the tax officials for checking. They concluded that he had overcharged by about 20 percent, mainly by too frequent visits. He still got back over $100,000. Oddly enough, nobody has complained very loudly at the president of ITT making $800,000 or so a year, and it seems to be OK for a hockey player or golfer to exceed a million dollars in a year for a lot fewer hours of work.

In Chapter 9 I mentioned my own experience in a company town in the late 1940s where, when medical insurance came in, my practice doubled although I did not encourage it. I did not mention the climax of the story, the only time in my life I have been fired from a job.

I was ordered to appear before a joint meeting of management and union to show why the medical plan was going broke. Although I protested that most of the money was being spent on visits to specialists in the big city (I had no control over this), the fact that I was earning $1,000 per month, more than the manager, was sufficient to damn me in their eyes. They seemed to expect that either I would see patients and not charge for my advice or I would turn patients away. As I refused to work for nothing and could not refuse to see a patient demanding treatment, their attitude was unfair, and I said so bluntly. The argument became extremely acrimonious and finally I said, "All right. So I make too much money. Then I'll work for a salary at union rates."

There was dead silence for a moment.

Finally the union leader spoke. "Work for a salary at union rates? You can't do that."

"Why not?" I said. "What's more, I'll take the minimum wage of a dollar an hour even though I'm the most skilled worker in the plant."

They looked puzzled.

A foreman spoke up. "There's got to be a gimmick somewhere."

"You're damn right," I exclaimed. "Union rules, that's the gimmick. As the only doctor in town, my contract states that I'm either on duty or on call twenty-four hours a day and seven days a week. By your own rules I must be paid full rates if I'm on call. At time and a half eight hours and double time after sixteen, plus double time on Saturday and Sunday, it comes to nearly $1,200 for a thirty-day month. Figure it out for yourselves and then figure what you'd have to pay me as a skilled worker at $3.00 per hour. And you say I'm making too much money!"

"Ah, but you're a doctor," the manager said. "That's different."

"To hell with you all," I said. "I've had it."

"Are you quitting?" the manager asked.

"No. If I quit I get nothing. If you fire me you have to pay me three months' notice and, by God, I'll make you glad to do it."

The rest is censored. Three months later I left, with an extra three months' salary.

That was in 1948. Recently in a letter to the *American Medical News* a doctor in California noted that a plumber in that state makes $14 or more per hour, plus overtime. At thirty-five hours per week he takes home $24,000 per year. He also gets retirement fund, paid vacation, life insurance, health insurance and other fringe benefits, none of which the private practitioner can have. The average work week of the California GP is sixty hours. The average annual net earnings are $36,000. At plumbers' rates, with say twenty hours counted as overtime (at time and a half only) he would make $51,900. I would think that a doctor is worth at least as much to the community as a plumber and yet people begrudge him equal remuneration for his hours of work.

It happens in other countries too. Recently in Australia there has been uproar because the GPs were increasing their fees. Amid a lot of snide remarks about the poor doctor making house calls in his Rolls Royce, the *Australian* newspaper published some very revealing statistics. The new fee for a basic consultation in the home was set by the Australian Medical Association at $7.35. Yet if a refrigerator mechanic were called to fix your machine, he would charge $7.00 for the first fifteen minutes. To fix an air-conditioner cost $14 per hour, which included traveling time. The doctor does not charge for that.

It is no wonder doctors get sour when they are subjected to so much criticism over their incomes. The hate can go both ways, and it is a very sad situation.

11

Everybody Knows About Freud

1. Nobody Dies, Nobody is Cured

In my days as a student there were three specialties that were considered safe bets for the unambitious who wanted a good living. The first was obstetrics because most babies will be born naturally and everyone is happy when they arrive. The second was dermatology because, as we put it, "Nobody dies and nobody is cured." The third was psychiatry for similar reasons and also because the treatment consisted mainly of talk. That is no longer true.

2. Who Can Afford It?

As a part of the Freudian school of psychiatry, psychoanalysis has been popular for a long time. It was fashionable for movie stars and other so-called eminent people to visit their analysts. Authors steeped in Freudian mythology made millions writing novels which the critics acclaimed for their deep psychological insights, mostly balderdash as far as I could see, and Freudian jargon cluttered up the language with terms such as complexes, fixations, the id, the unconscious, the ego and superego and so on. None of these concepts was subject to proof as we generally understand it. We had to take Freud's ideas on faith, as we do religion. Before the biochemistry boom there was no system of psychiatric treatment except witchcraft. Since that was so, analysis became popular. There was only one trouble: it cost too much in money and time.

My son-in-law is a psychiatrist and my eldest daughter, his wife, is a general practitioner. As part of his training he has undergone analysis and she has had it too, since their lives are linked together. There is no doubt in their minds that it has helped them to understand and cope with life's problems, and, having watched them over the years, I agree. However, it has taken several hours a week, has gone on for years and is not over yet. Even for them it is expensive, since the analyst must be paid for his time. For the ordinary person it is simply not feasible.

There have been studies in the last few years claiming that analysis is no better than TLC (tender loving care) and I am inclined to agree. The difficulty again arises: who has the time to give TLC to all those who need it? The clergy are now beginning to work closely with psychiatrists and general practitioners, and this may well be their field of greatest usefulness now that Christianity and the other religions seem to be losing their grip on people. We should work on it.

3. Happiness Is a Pill

At times in recent years it looked as if the materialists were right and man was nothing but a complicated series of biochemical and biophysical reactions. Love and hate, kindness and cruelty, truth and falsehood all were said to depend on the state of our enzymes. When we read about a cat becoming terrified of a mouse after being given a certain chemical, or of lions cuddling up to lambs (to stretch the point a bit), we began to wonder if this could be true. The great biochemical boom was on and Miltown became a household word.

There is no doubt that there are definite biochemical changes in neuropsychiatric disease. In depressive psychosis there appears to be a lack of or inability to use norepinephrine, a substance which controls drive, activity level, exploratory behavior, alertness and aggressive reactions. Drugs such as amphetamine (dexedrine) seem to prevent norepinephrine being stored away in the nerve cell where it is not used, and so, when given dexedrine, the patient feels better. In schizophrenia, among other effects there seems to be a blockage of nerve mechanisms which use serotonin, a substance that is involved in the control of mood. This blockage can be removed by drugs such as trifluoperazine. However, an overdose can cause a type of muscular restlessness or even simulate Parkinson's disease. The actions of these drugs are usually complex and can be dangerous, as I have mentioned elsewhere. Nevertheless, the pressure on the doctor to use them is tremendous. "I need a pill to sleep, doctor," is easily followed by "I feel dopey. Can't you give me something to pep me up?" And so the patient bounces from barbiturate to dexedrine and the drug manufacturers get rich.

The bad part is that all this manipulation does not get at the root causes of psychiatric disease but merely ameliorates symptoms. Are we really just biochemical bombs or is there something beyond our chemistry?

A very disturbing aspect of this happiness-is-a-pill concept was reported in the *Washington Post* on June 30, 1970, and on July 4, on the Huntley-Brinkley television show. They announced that doctors in Omaha, Nebraska, were giving hundreds of children so-called behavior-modification drugs to "make them behave better in school."

Certain children are hyperactive or fidgety and disrupt classes.

Perhaps they react compulsively to external stimuli that others can ignore. We do not know the reason, but we do know that they can be quieted by using drugs such as tranquillizers and, paradoxically, the amphetamines, which seem to block out some stimuli, such as fatigue and hunger, which are unsettling. Antidepressants are also used for children made irritable and restless by neurotic depression.

The dangers of this approach are several. If the doctor is experienced in handling these drugs, we can probably rule out causing addiction. We cannot rule out misdiagnosis. The physician often has to depend on teachers' reports since he himself cannot spend much time with each child. What one teacher would consider abnormal behavior another might dismiss as merely boisterousness. Much depends on the amount of harassment the teacher can endure. Some children are definitely abnormal, but they should be treated only under proper psychiatric supervision for long periods of time.

There are other problems in control by pills. One is the risk of contributing to the drug culture. Another is that the drugged child can hardly learn self-control and is deprived of the chance to acquire insight into his own problems. Finally, there are the legal aspects. Children have rights, as recent court cases show, and what teachers consider disruptive may not be illegal. Interference with those rights, no matter how well-intentioned, is interference with each person's constitutional liberties.

The amount of mental illness in the youth of our nation is growing. According to Dr. Stanley F. Yolles, Director of the National Institute of Mental Health, in 1967 youngsters were being admitted to mental hospitals in numbers *seven times their share of the total population*. Between 1960 and 1965 the number of U.S. psychiatrists, psychologists and other mental-health workers rose 44 percent, but it was not enough. The *Lancet*, of Great Britain, on November 20, 1971, in an article entitled "Aid for the Adolescent," stated that doctors were unable to cope with the psychological problems of the young in Great Britain. The juggernaut we have built is crushing our children.

We had better watch how we handle these psychological problems. We may find that the Brave New World of Aldous Huxley is coming up on the horizon. 1984 is not far away.

4. Drinks and Drugs

In 1970 Dr. Daniel Friedman, Director of the American Psychiatric Association's task force on drug abuse, said that the number-one drug problem was alcohol. It was the cause of at least 86,000 deaths each year. There were between 7 and 9 million alcoholics in the United States and in 1969 drinking drivers and pedestrians accounted for 30,000 automobile deaths. As I wrote this I had just come from the Outpatient Department in Lae. A Melanesian driver, drunk, had overturned a passenger truck full of people. There were four dead and twenty injured. I saw similar cases in Africa, where alcohol and sex are the main sources of amusement, especially in the shanty towns near big cities.

A less serious problem, although it gets more publicity because we drinkers can look down our noses at the offenders, is drug addiction. There may be 300,000 heroin addicts in the United States. I have it from a senior Army public health officer that the problem in returned Vietnam veterans has been exaggerated. There were supposed to be 100,000 addicts in New York in 1971 and 1,205 narcotic-related deaths, of which 237 were teenagers. I do not think anyone knows how many marijuana smokers there are.

The problem in both alcohol and heroin is addiction. Some researchers believe that there are permanent metabolic changes due to these substances that induce an appetite for the same drug after its use is discontinued. Simple observation of ex-smokers who crave a fag for many months and of alcoholics who go back years after kicking the habit certainly supports the idea that the desire for some drugs lasts a long time. Whether it is an incurable biochemical urge or amenable to psychotherapy nobody can say. In this era of biochemically induced moods the border between organic disease and psychoses is obscure. In March 1971, in the *American Journal of Psychiatry*, a study by Drs. Shuckit, Goodwin and Winokur reported on children of alcoholic parents raised by non-drinking foster parents. When they grew up they were six times as likely to be problem drinkers as others from parents who were not alcoholics. The doctors stated that genetics may have more influence than environment in the evolution of the problem drinker.

The medical profession has not come to agreement on how addiction can be overcome. Treatments range from complete abstention and psychotherapy, through blocking drugs that negate the kick of heroin or cause nausea in intake of alcohol, to the British system of making cheap heroin readily available in well-controlled clinics. In America we have the new methadone treatment, which, in effect, substitutes for heroin a less dangerous, cheaper but still addictive drug. Obviously we do not have the right answer yet. My personal view is that once the fantastic profit is taken out of the illicit drug trade by letting doctors prescribe for addicts as the British do, we will have a better chance of clearing up the mess. As for alcohol, the sheer size of the problem makes it a public health matter. We have to approach alcoholism as a disease and not a crime. When we do, and get the community to work with us, we may be on the way to beating it. There is no instant solution. As long as two thirds of the adults in the United States drink and think teetotalers are a bit odd, we will be handicapped in treating alcoholics.

5. Anybody Can Give Advice

In all the furor about the doctor shortage one of the suggestions has been to separate the doctor from the patient by a screen of tests and tiers of less qualified people. The idea is that only the seriously ill or problem cases need to see him. Screening out the "worried-well" and the "not-so-sick" is a good idea in theory but is not fully tested in practice. A major problem is how to handle the psychological aspects of illness. The mere fact of seeing and talking to the doctor, the person who "knows how to take care of me," is a large part of the GP's treatment.

Recently in Australia there has been a lot of argument about the disappearing GPs. Whatever the cause—and I refer you to Chapter 5—there have been numerous suggestions on how to solve the difficulties engendered by their disappearance. In the *Australian* newspaper of February 24, 1972, two young and confident gentlemen put forth a solution. One, Dr. Vance Gledhill, a computer expert and researcher, said, "The GP is something that went out with raccoon coats and button-up boots. He is a luxury we can't afford any more." Thereby he showed a lamentable lack of knowledge, since GPs were still in the majority twenty years after the coats and boots were banished to the attic. He went on to say that the patient would fill out a questionnaire *at home* which would then go to a central computer for analysis and storage. He stated that it could diagnose patients better than eight doctors who looked at the same questionnaire. The computer was right in 70 percent of cases and the doctors only in 42 percent. How he knew that the computer was right and the doctors wrong is something he failed to explain.

According to this expert, straightforward illnesses did not need the doctor. All one had to do was follow the computer's advice. As for the other functions of the GPs, he said that they were ill-equipped anyway to perform social medicine and "We have to break down the barriers in Australia against psychiatrists." He added that under computer medicine, doctors would be protected from hypochondriacs for the first time. "We will be able to screen the sick from the worried-well." Where all the psychiatrists, who cost a lot more than GPs, would come from this computer expert did not say.

I have paraphrased this article at length to show that anyone can give advice, but not all of it is good. The young man was very sure of himself, but I wonder how many offices full of GPs' patients he has had to handle. I wonder too, if he has a wife, how she will react when her child is ill to sitting down at home to tick off answers to dozens of questions and then being told, when she drives to the clinic, that she does not need to see the doctor.

It is said that over half the female patients seen by doctors in the United States are psychiatric problems. One half of all hospital beds in the United States are devoted to the care of psychiatric patients. The situation has been greatly improved by the new biochemical psychiatry in that previously troublesome patients are now easier to handle and neurotics can be tranquillized or pepped up. The result, according to the Veterans Administration in a report in *Military Medicine*, August 1971, is that the use of such drugs enables the VA to treat twice as many psychiatric patients as previously, without an increase in hospital beds. To me this is an indication of how many were neglected or attended at home before they could be drugged into a more normal frame of mind. However, as I said above, this does not get at the root of the trouble, which is probably the life style of the patients and of the culture in which they live.

In spite of our optimistic computer expert, it will be quite impossible to train enough psychiatrists to take care of the mental ailments of all the people. We cannot afford it, in any case. A minimal psychiatric consultation is much more time-consuming and therefore more expensive than that for most organic disease. Like analysis, treatment can go on for years and the patient may never be cured but relapse at intervals for the rest of his life. It may be possible, after he has seen the doctor, to turn him over to a clergyman or a social psychologist. Attempts are now being made to use kindly, intelligent laymen (some doctors say preferably with no psychiatric training so they will not have some half-baked theories on treatment) as therapists. What that comes down to is TLC again, a commodity the whole world can use. In the village of Gheel in Holland something of the sort has been going on for many years, with psychiatric cases being boarded out to families that have come to know how to handle them. It could be that the mere feeling of belonging, to a family or a group, is all that most of our neurotics need. It is a feeling that has been lost in our modern society with its broken-up family structure.

In the undeveloped nations where there may be one psychiatrist to a million people, little can be done beyond TLC. However, after years of attempted suppression by missionaries and governments, witchcraft is getting another chance. To readers of the pulps, witchcraft conjures up visions of a leaping devil doctor pointing the bone at some terrified victim who is then killed or dies of fright. This was true to some extent in the past, but today the *nganga*, as the Bantu witch doctor is called, is mostly a herbalist and faith healer. He understands his tribesmen as the white doctor cannot do and, being a shrewd judge of character, he can play on their emotions and alter their moods. In short, he can handle many psychological problems quite well and, as he gives out his herbs, he satisfies the desire to "get a prescription" which I mentioned before. Some of the experienced Western-trained doctors in Africa have a working relationship with the local *nganga* on which patients each should handle and they refer them to each other. It seems to be a better arrangement than competition and jealousy.

6. Into the Never-Never Land

Mention of the *nganga* brings me back to the subjects I mentioned in Chapter 3. I refer to acupuncture, yoga, hypnosis and the possibilities in thought control (as seen by our newfound ability to control the alpha waves of the brain) and perhaps thought transference or telepathy. It is already well known that our mental state strongly influences our physical condition. I remember a husband with a proved stomach ulcer who improved when he took my suggestion and got away from his nagging wife for a while into a restful atmosphere. That is a crude example. We need much more research into these rather nebulous areas. It may eventually be a far more profitable road than the pill path.

I once met a surgeon who had removed a patient's thyroid gland while the patient was hypnotized. I saw a dentist work on a hypnotized doctor's gums and the patient felt no pain. I watched another hypnotized doctor control his heartbeat under suggestion. Nowadays, using the biofeedback technique of brain-wave control, patients with heart disease have been taught to stop irregular heartbeats and speed up or slow their hearts by mental control (not under hypnosis). Rats have been taught to control intestinal contractions mentally and Dr. Neal Miller of Rockefeller University has taught a rat to blush one ear and blanch the other at the same time. The yogis of India were said to be able to cleanse their gastrointestinal tract merely by thinking about it. The time may come when we learn to do the same. As Dr. Miller said in 1971, "We are now able to regard the activities of our internal organs as behavior in the same sense as the movements of our hands and fingers are behavior."

Mental control of our viscera is in its early stages. Control of our emotions, or irrational fears and anxieties might follow as we learn more. However, I feel that to achieve true mind control will require a totally different attitude toward life. It will require hours of contemplation, if the success achieved by Hindu mystics is any criterion. Of course, we may find electromechanical or drug short cuts (plenty of people are trying that now) to the control we desire. That would be in line with our present life style. If the end result should be a nation of mentally satisfied materialists, then I want no part of it. While the world dies I won't feel like laughing.

To my mind, psychiatric illness is to the rest of disease as the underwater iceberg is to what we see. If we compare the percentages of medical workers in psychiatry to those in the other branches of medicine, we see that, once again, medicine is misdirected. Far more attention is given to the physical diseases, probably because we can get at them with our treatments; we know their causes and their cures. Yet even they are overlaid with psychological problems, and the sick mind can cause physical changes.

Psychiatric disease is increasing. In the VA report I mentioned above, it was stated that in the four years before 1960 the number of veterans seeking treatment in the VA psychiatric clinics doubled. T. R. Harrison *et al*, in *Principles of Internal Medicine*, fourth edition, state, "As a clinical syndrome the anxiety state outranks all other diagnostic problems in general medicine." They quote Willoughby, who said anxiety is "the most prominent mental characteristic of Occidental civilization." We are trying to control it these days with our drugs, but that is treating symptoms and not getting at the cause. We need to know much more about our minds and how they work. If we are to continue with any research, there, it seems to me, is the greatest hope for the future.

12
Civilization Is Killing Me

1. Whodunit?

A PECULIARITY OF PEOPLE is that most of them do not like to think or do not believe that they are animals. They believe that either God or evolution has somehow raised them onto a higher plane where they are not subject to the natural laws governing the rest of the animal kingdom. They are wrong. It may also turn out that social evolution is a chimera, if we are to believe naturalists like Konrad Lorenz and Desmond Morris and the dramatist Robert Ardrey. In years to come, when the people problem is at its height, we are likely to find out.

It takes an elementary knowledge of evolution to realize that if man remained essentially unchanged in his physical characteristics for thousands of years until the end of the eighteenth century, he is unlikely to have changed perceptibly since that time. Without a great mutation—and we have no evidence that one has occurred—man is the same today as he was at the start of the industrial revolution. That revolution changed our way of life and I intend in this chapter to show what it has done to our bodies. We cannot blame the consequences on an act of God or natural causes. If you ask me, "Whodunit?" I can only say, "We did."

2. The Great Plague

If the average person read in the papers that plague had returned to the United States, killing more than 2,000 people every day and hospitalizing thousands more, he would be terribly worried. With his neighbors he would line up for inoculations, demand antibiotics, take his family off to an isolated summer cottage and quite possibly get into a state of panic.

Arteriosclerosis does kill and cripple that many. Well over half the deaths in the United States are due to it. It is a plague of sorts, but we take it more or less for granted as the normal end of the human race. Most people in the civilized world, including doctors, are unaware that in other countries the disease is almost unknown.

For nearly seven years I lived and worked in Kenya and Malawi. I performed or watched hundreds of autopsies on both young and old people, mostly blacks. In all that time, except for one black man, the only fatal cases of arteriosclerotic heart disease or stroke that I saw were in white people or East Indians. Furthermore, on examining the arteries of the blacks, I was amazed at how little arteriosclerosis there was in them. Old black men, dead in accidents or for other causes, had arteries that a thirty-year-old American would be glad to have. Some of the blacks died of arterial aneurysms due to syphilis, but this was rare. In other words, the vascular disease that kills our civilized people was not affecting the uncivilized black man.

I say uncivilized black man because the modern American Negro gets arteriosclerosis. In West Africa, where most of the American slaves originated, the disease is still rare, so it is not a matter of inheritance. In South Africa, where the whites have one of the highest rates of arteriosclerotic heart disease in the world, the rural Bantu is immune, living in the same area. It is not, therefore, a climatic or geographical thing. It is simply due to the way we live.

Billions of dollars and uncounted hours have been spent in investigating this disease. Most of the research has been into the hydrodynamics of blood flow in arteries or into the complicated interactions of biochemical substances in general metabolism or in the vessels themselves. Much advice has been given about lowering the blood pressure and lessening the amount of cholesterol in the blood. Lack of exercise and mental stress have been blamed. Drugs have been prescribed to alter the metabolic processes to prevent the lipid deposits in the inner lining of arteries which eventually lead to ulceration and closure of the vessels. Specially equipped ambulances are now cruising the streets keeping flagging hearts going until they reach the hospital. Surgeons do transplants of vessels or even hearts or cut out damaged areas. If the brain is affected, surgery is done to relieve the pressure caused by hemorrhages. Since we cannot yet repair damaged nerve pathways or induce nerve cells to regenerate, we spend colossal amounts of money and effort keeping paralyzed people alive and attempting to reeducate nerves and muscles so that some return of function can be achieved. And still the slaughter goes on. If he knew, the untutored savage, squatting by his fire, would laugh derisively at supposedly superior civilized man dying by his own hand as surely as if he were wielding a knife.

It is all preventable. I am quite certain of it. And we already know how. Researchers in laboratories have been confirming what observers in the field, in the tropics, have been seeing for years. The trouble lies in getting doctors and patients to believe it strongly enough to make drastic changes in their life style. It does not matter that we do not know the exact cause or how prevention works. We use many procedures and drugs without really understanding their mechanisms. Then why wait? All we have to do is to eat what the savage eats and live (with some obvious reservations regarding hygiene) as he does. Our specialists try to tell us that it is undernourished poor people who are free of arteriosclerosis. This is nonsense, as I have mentioned in Chapter 2. Many of these people are far fitter than we are, in spite of their parasites and, to us, inadequate and unpalatable diets.

Through millions of years our bodies evolved so that when we lived on natural foods in balanced amounts, such as we might obtain by hunting or gathering plants or by primitive agriculture, then we would be healthy. Here, of course, I am not concerned with the infectious diseases, parasites and so on which killed ancient man. Medical science took the right path when it discovered how to eliminate these pests. It went wrong when it failed to realize what man was doing to himself by becoming "civilized."

3. Take a Deep Breath

Today, not only are we killing ourselves with our teeth—i.e., by faulty diets—we are also killing ourselves by breathing: by breathing polluted air and tobacco smoke. It is already quite obvious, except perhaps to those who work for the polluters or tobacco companies, that we are in serious trouble. Lung cancer is now a major disease in civilized countries. Bronchitis and emphysema of the lungs are responsible for much of the morbidity in older people in smog-ridden cities. The death rate from chronic lung disease in Great Britain is much higher than in Norway with its cleaner air. About 20 percent of adult British males have chronic cough and phlegm production. In Norway it is 6.1 percent. In America it approaches the British figure.

The relationship of tobacco to cancer is not clear. The Rhodesian tobacco farmer, one of the heaviest smokers in the world, gets less lung cancer than the Englishman who lives in London and smokes the same amount. One theory is that smoking stops the action of the cilia of the bronchial cells from moving mucus to where it can be coughed out or swallowed and this allows carcinogens in the dust of polluted cities to come into prolonged contact with the cells. Eventually cancer begins. The Rhodesian escapes to some extent because he smokes in an otherwise unpolluted atmosphere. Whatever the reason, lung cancer is a disease mainly of our own making, and so are bronchitis and emphysema. If we cleared up the air and cut out smoking, they would probably disappear in a generation.

We may have to give up our cars as well as our fags if we want to be really safe. Back in the 1950s Dr. Charles Larsen, the well-known Tacoma pathologist, pointed out the dangers from asbestos dust in the Navy Yards on Puget Sound. During the frantic shipbuilding of the war era, workers were busy putting asbestos insulation on ships' pipes, and later some of them began to die of a cancerous growth called a mesothelioma. It had been known for a long time that asbestos fibers were very irritating to the lungs, and attempts were made to reduce the exposure to safe levels. Overexposure produced a gradual fibrosis of the lung tissues that cut down the area available for gas exchange, and the patient gradually suffocated. Now it seemed that he could also die of cancer. The so-called safe levels were not safe enough. It now appears that 38 percent of those working in "safe levels" for more than twenty years have the fibrosis and there is no known way to stop its progress. How much exposure is dangerous we do not really know, and that is why we might have to give up our automobiles. There is now an increasing amount of asbestos dust in the air of our cities, brought about, no doubt, by the stoplight race. Every time we slam on our brakes a minute amount of asbestos floats off them into the air to join the lead fumes and other noxious gases we breathe. Obviously, new devices for filtering exhausts will not filter out the asbestos and so we will not be able to sit back and relax after all. For my money, we should bring back the horse. At least we can use his emissions to grow roses to counteract the smell.

Where doctors go wrong is in not making enough fuss about air pollution, and in their own human frailty in continuing to smoke and drive gas-eating monsters, which sets a bad example to their patients. There is hope, however, in the new laws concerning automobile emissions and air pollution, if they can be rigidly enforced. There is also hope that a harmless cigarette will be produced for those who cannot stop the habit.

As I began writing this I found something else for us to worry about. In January 1972 it was reported that Dr. Milne, a chemist in the National Heart and Lung Institute of the United States, had found chemicals from plastics in the bloodstreams of 86 out of 100 laboratory workers and patients in the hospital where he worked. These phthalate esters, as they are called, are used in making polyvinyl chloride, which is used to make car upholstery, blood-transfusion bags, water bottles, floor coverings, food wraps and even insecticides. In short, they are all around us. Dr. Milne found from 10 to 30 parts per million in human blood serum. Apparently they are soluble in blood, milk and fats, and also escape into the air to be breathed in.

Nobody yet knows if they are harmful. The amounts may seem small, but it takes only five parts per million of DDT to be dangerous, so who can say? An official of the White House Council on Environmental Quality was quoted as saying, "I know this is going to be a significant future issue. It's potentially our next bad one."

I hope, thirty years from now, that quote will not be the epitaph for Homo civilizatus.

4. Bulk and Bowels

In the Western world today cancer of the large bowel is one of the commoner tumors. There is also a condition called diverticulosis in which tiny pockets form in the walls of the large intestine rather like a blowout in a bicycle tube. These numerous little pockets become infected and sometimes perforate. Another disease we get is regional ileitis, which gave President Eisenhower so much pain, and, in the large bowel, ulcerative colitis, which is so distressing that long sections of the gut may have to be removed. Much research has been done on these diseases and special bland low-residue diets have been prescribed for the sufferers. Our doctors could hardly be more wrong.

In my years in Africa I never saw any of these diseases in Africans. They did get anal cancers, but some of those were probably due to infestation with the worm called bilharzia or schistosomiasis, which lays its eggs in rectum or bladder and causes incalculable suffering throughout the African continent. My friend Mr. Dennis Burkitt (English surgeons are not called doctor), whose name has been given to the dreadful tumors he described from Uganda, has gathered information on intestinal diseases from all over Africa. From his own experience and from these data he confirms my observations. The African does not suffer from these intestinal diseases. He does get typhoid and tuberculosis of the gut, but these are infectious conditions.

Why is this so? According to Dennis, with great difficulty he persuaded a group of English boarding-school boys to eat certain marker substances with their meals and collect the feces in plastic bags. He did the same with a similar group of Uganda native schoolboys. The results were quite astonishing. The Bantu boys had more frequent and bulkier stools and the markers came through at least twice as fast as with the English boys. It appears from this and from laboratory investigations into pressure changes in the gut that high-residue, largely vegetable diets, as eaten by the Ugandans, are easier to propel through the intestine. The small, constipated stool of the English boys took longer and was more difficult to move. The result, he believes, is that the intestinal wall gives way after years of such pressures and diverticula form. Also, as the stools are in more prolonged contact with the cells of the lining wall, carcinogens in them have more chance of causing disease.

If this theory is true, and I believe it could be, our diet is definitely bad for us and treatment by low-residue diets only makes the diverticulitis worse. There are now a few papers being published on the use of high-residue diets in Europeans with diverticulitis. The results seem good. Perhaps we are now on the right path to treatment and, if people will listen, to prevention.

As an appendix to this section I wish to discuss that organ. (Please excuse the pun.) Appendicitis was not commonly diagnosed in our great-grandfathers' day. I am quite sure that, like arteriosclerosis, it would have been recorded by the great clinicians of the time whenever present. It is rare today in Africans and the people of New Guinea, although it seems to be increasing. I feel that this is another of the benefits of civilization and is probably dietary. There is some evidence that it has decreased in the West since the end of the Second World War. Nobody is quite sure why. One idea is that clearing up infections elsewhere with antibiotics may prevent infection of the appendix. They may also cause appendicitis to subside before operative removal becomes necessary.

Some say that removal of tonsils, once popular, exposed the appendix to infection. As both organs are part of the lymphoreticular protection system this seems possible.

5. Sugar! Lumps or Sticks?

Diabetes is a relatively rare condition among most undeveloped peoples. An exception is the Pima Indians of Arizona, who have a rate of diabetes ten to fifteen times that of the general population of the United States. With them it could be hereditary. I do not know what they eat.

In other areas where refined sugars and carbohydrates form a good portion of the diet, diabetes is common. So is arteriosclerosis, and some physicians blame refined carbohydrates as the cause. In Durban, South Africa, the East Indians eat much carbohydrate, mostly refined, and they have one of the highest rates of diabetes in the world. Their poorer relatives in India, on a diet of more basic carbohydrate, are not plagued with the disease. This does not prove the point, of course, but it seems that, while it requires good teeth, it might be safer to get one's sugar by chewing the cane than by taking white granules from a packet. Recently it has been claimed that keeping fit lessens the requirement for antidiabetic drugs in the sufferers. Perhaps we should go out and cut our own cane or dig up our own sugar beets.

6. Fair, Fat, Forty, Female

The history of disease is fascinating and gives some insight into the results of man's interference with nature and the consequences of changes in his habits. In the eighteenth century, bladder stones were fairly common and bladder colic was a very painful and disabling condition. As there was no anesthesia other than alcohol and perhaps opium, surgeons became famous for the skill and speed with which they could plunge their knife up through the screaming victim's perineum into the bladder and flip out the stone with a long finger. Nowadays bladder stones are rare. We have gallstone colic instead.

It is estimated that 15 to 20 million Americans have gallstones. How much ill health these cause by interfering with normal bile flow nobody can say. When I was on the wards I learned that if I saw a female, fair, fat and about forty with abdominal pain and indigestion, I was probably dealing with a case of cholelithiasis—i.e., stones in the gallbladder. Aspiring surgeons graduated from hernias and appendicitis to operations on the gallbladder, which were much more difficult. Pathologists became adept at describing the changes in the removed gallbladder. They still are, but not in Africa. Aside from a rare case of soft pigment stones that I might see at an autopsy, I do not recall more than a handful of cases of gallbladder disease in Africans, and jaundice was more likely due to hemolytic anemia than to obstruction by a stone in the bile duct as it commonly is in America. Thus it appears that we can add gallstones to the roster of diseases of civilization.

7. Legs are for Locomotion, Not Looks

Varicose veins are not nearly as common in Africa as they are in America. The African walks or bicycles while the American drives. This may be the reason for the difference—better skin and muscle tone and so better circulation. The difference is important for another reason. After operations, especially in older people, one of the feared complications is thrombophlebitis, which is inflammation and clot formation in veins, usually of the legs or pelvis, and more common in those with bad circulation. If a large clot breaks loose, it may go up through the heart into the pulmonary arteries and block the circulation to the lungs. This is called a pulmonary embolus and it kills many Americans each year. I have yet to see one in an African. They seem to come through surgical operations without this complication. I am quite sure they escape and we are at risk because of our life style. I suspect it is because they are a lot fitter than we are.

We should be using our legs much more than we do. They provide us with the easiest way of keeping fit. Lifting barbells or doing pushups in the apartment may give us muscles that look good on the beach, but it is recognized that really life-saving exercise must cause the heart and lungs to work hard for relatively long periods of time if we are to keep them in tone. Walking at a fast pace several miles a day or jogging for at least a mile and a half will do it. The fast fifty-yard dash for a bus is likely to do more harm than good. This does not mean that previously sedentary individuals should suddenly get out and run hard. That might kill them.

Just how poor our condition is was brought home to us in President Eisenhower's term of office, when a study showed that American schoolchildren were not nearly as fit as the Europeans. We should not have been surprised. Most kids nowadays sit in the stands screaming their heads off as their athletic idols prance around the field. They develop strong vocal chords, as any father listening to rock records will testify, but little else.

We have almost forgotten that blow to our pride way back in

the 1950s, but we can take satisfaction from knowing that now it is the Europeans' turn. In a study by the Physical Culture Research Institute of Prague, Czechoslovakia, reported in the *Medical Tribune*, May 1971, a comparison of Tunisian and Czechoslovakian children was made. The children were about twelve years old. In Tunisia they came from poorer families but with an adequate living standard, and from privileged families with boys in a Tunisian private school. The Czech boys were average for their nation. They were much taller and heavier than the poor Tunisians, with the rich Tunisians in between. The poor Tunisians were much fitter and stronger than the others. They got much more exercise and were not as fat as the wealthier boys. Dr. Paizkova, who was one of the researchers, commented, "The huge increases in height and weight we have noted in children in all industrialized countries, especially since the war, may not be the most desirable trend in children's health care." He added, "Let's not make the mistake of exporting obesity and lowered physical fitness along with technological advantages."

When I was a paratrooper during the Korean War we did not want anyone over two hundred pounds in weight. Such men dropped faster, hit the ground harder and might get hurt. They were also bigger targets, ate more and could shoot no better. When we went on maneuvers we used to leave the big boys behind to play American football for the Division. It was the only use we had for them. The American public loves these enormous men in spite of the fact that the lighter, smaller fellow with the low blood pressure seems to live longest. Perhaps it is because the spectators can make a hero of someone as blimpish in build as they are.

Speaking of blood pressure, it has been considered for years that, as a man aged, so his blood pressure would go up. One formula was 100 plus age for normal systolic pressure. It was axiomatic that with this rise in pressure there would be a greater risk of developing strokes, heart failure and kidney damage. Arteriosclerosis is linked to the rising pressure too, but, not to get too involved, let me add that obesity and poor condition also play a part. At any rate, it is certain that rises in blood pressure are associated with shortening of the life span. Some researchers say that the tendency to hypertension may be inherited.

Here again I am inclined to think that civilization is at fault. In primitive peoples such as the New Guinea native and in many rural African tribesmen the blood pressure does not rise appreciably with age and strokes are practically unknown, except in rare cases of malignant hypertension. Yet hypertension occurs early and in a higher percentage of blacks in the United States and Panama than in whites. Surely it must be due to a change in their life style as compared with their African cousins.

It is my guess that the African, on the average, is more fit and leads a mentally more relaxed life than American blacks do. This is certainly true compared to the white man. I only wish we could compare the hard-working mule-driving, corn-eating Southern Negro sharecropper of 50 to 100 years ago with his car-riding, beef-eating great-grandson. I believe the older generation was less subject to high blood pressure and its consequences.

8. Two Plus Two Equals Five

Iatrogenic disease—i.e., disease caused by the doctor—has been known for many years and varies from psychiatric upsets to simple vomiting brought on, for example, by giving an ergotamine preparation for migraine. Never before has the doctor had such a profusion of drugs to use, and it is now well recognized that when he uses them, he had better be sure the effect will not add up to more than he bargained for. The problem is one of complicated biochemical linkages and we are far from a full understanding of it. It gets worse when we realize that there are numerous genetic variations in the way each person's biochemical constitution works, so that the old saying "One man's meat is another man's poison" can come true.

Let me give examples. Certain Mediterranean peoples, some blacks and others cannot eat the broad bean (fava bean) so beloved of British gardeners. If they do, it triggers a breakdown of their red blood cells. This is due to a genetically determined deficiency of an enzyme called glucose 6PD. Every year a few Sardinian children die from eating these beans. The same hemolytic effect can occur in these deficient people following treatment with aspirin, certain sulfonamides and other drugs. These are examples of drugs acting on the enzyme systems of the body.

Drugs also interact with each other in the body. The sedative phenobarbital somehow stimulates the metabolic breakdown of other drugs given at the same time, thus lessening their effect. The coumarin derivatives used to prevent abnormal blood clotting—e.g., after a heart attack—are broken down faster when the patient receives an ordinary dose of phenobarbital. Thus higher doses of the anticoagulant must be used. The reverse is true when aspirin or tetracycline is given—the coumarin persists longer in the blood, and so overdosage can become a problem, as too much anticoagulant can lead to serious bleeding.

There are other dangers. Some analgesics (to relieve pain) are believed to cause inflammation in the kidney. Ordinarily we accept the small risk to gain the pain-killing power. But what if the kidney is already sick? Or what if the liver is moderately damaged and cannot detoxify a certain drug in a reasonable time? The effect of the drug then continues much longer than intended, with possibly serious effects.

Books have now been written about these interactions of drugs with themselves and the body. No doctor can know all the possible combinations. He can minimize them by using as few drugs for as short a time as possible, if the patient does not object to a bit more discomfort. A recent study at Johns Hopkins Hospital by Dr. Cluff and his associates is pertinent. Of patients in the hospital who were receiving from 6 to 10 drugs, 4.2 percent reported some adverse reaction such as nausea, vomiting, skin rash, renal difficulty and so on. Of those getting 11 to 15 drugs, 24.2 percent had reactions. Of those who had 16 to 20 drugs, 40 percent had reactions, and 45 percent getting more than 20 drugs had reactions. About 4 percent of all patients admitted to the general medical service were admitted *because of* an adverse drug reaction, and before they got out again, 30 percent of these poor souls had had another drug reaction. And this was in one of the finest teaching hospitals in the world!

9. The Guy's a Quack

At the risk of annoying my colleagues, I have to report that not all iatrogenic disease is due to unexpected interreactions of drugs and enzymes. Some of it is due to patient pressure for medication, but some is due to careless prescribing by the doctors themselves.

In a recent investigation by Dr. Harry F. Dowling, an authority on infectious diseases and drug therapy, it was reported after surveying 85,000 patients' charts that there was a justifiable reason for the use of antibiotics in only 54 percent of them. He also reported that in one hospital, in a series of operations for hernia, 32 percent of the patients were given antibiotics to prevent infection. In hernia operations done properly, there should be no infection. The patients were therefore subjected to needless risk and expense. Studying hernia operations in different hospitals, he found that the number of patients getting antibiotics varied from 3 to 82 percent. Clearly, someone is prescribing improperly.

Patient pressure is a real problem, as I know from my years as a GP. Many times doctors will give an antibiotic for a common cold, knowing that it will not destroy the virus, because the patient insists and will go to another doctor if he does not get what he wants. In the old days one could write a prescription in Latin and hope to fool the demanding patient. Nowadays Latin is not used and that subterfuge is gone. To be fair, there is some justification for antibiotics in virus conditions if there is a danger of secondary bacterial invasion and the patient is at home, not under close supervision.

Surveys in North Carolina, Ontario and Nova Scotia have shown that far too many general practitioners are guilty of poor work in both diagnosis and treatment, at least in the opinions of the specialists who did the investigations. Examples are the prescribing of penicillin for ordinary colds; treating anemia by "shotgun" prescriptions instead of making the exact diagnosis; prescribing various drugs for organic disease when the patient's troubles were emotional, and so on. In the hands of such men, modern methods can be dangerous.

I cannot justify this. I can only say that the same is true of politics, the law, business, science, engineering and the trades. Perhaps we are all bewildered by the complexities of the civilization we have built. It can kill us in more ways than one—the politician with his "brinkmanship," the soldiers with their H-bombs, the businessmen and engineers with pollution, the tradesmen with defective workmanship. The doctor has plenty of company.

13

The People Problem

1. Cuddle Up a Little Closer

THE POPULATION BOMB, as Dr. Paul R. Ehrlich calls it, is talked about so much these days that there should be little left to say. However, certain aspects of the problem as seen from a doctor's viewpoint might be worth exploring. People are a doctor's business and business has never boomed so much before.

The mere presence of people, healthy or not, creates problems. The city of São Paulo, Brazil, is reported to be the fastest-growing in the world. Every year 300,000 people flock into it, mostly to the slums. Half of the city's people are without running water and 70 percent are in areas with inadequate sewerage. There are 24,000 factories, God knows how many cars, and the pollution problems are appalling. It is a medical officer's nightmare. It is also a schoolmaster's migraine and a policeman's purgatory, but these problems are outside my scope.

As most readers know, crowding on the scale seen in São Paulo, Rio and Calcutta makes transmission of disease much easier. Cholera almost got into Calcutta in the recent Indo-Pakistan war.

Among the equally crowded Pakistani refugees in camps it killed thousands. Pneumonic plague, if it ever started in those rat-infested slums, would kill millions in a hurry. Whether that would be a disaster or a disguised blessing depends on your viewpoint. Influenza could strike again and, with inadequate medical attention allowing secondary infections to take hold, could kill as many as in 1918-20.

All this we know. There is one aspect of this crowding that could upset all our calculations. It may never happen, but if it does, we have no defense.

For hundreds of years it has been known that some animal species behave peculiarly when they become too numerous in an area. The march of the lemmings to the sea is the classic example. The sudden disappearance of rabbits and other rodents from the north country of Canada where in previous years they were numerous may be another instance. Some naturalists believe from field experience and laboratory experiments that this is a universal law. Each species needs a minimum space between individuals in which to live, and when the number in a given area exceeds the limit, trouble begins. The animals become irritable; they fight, even male and female; they perform unnatural sex acts, become cannibals, commit suicide. They do this even though abundant food and water are present where they live or are supplied in the laboratory tests. Eventually they stop breeding or females abort. The population drops far below the usual maintenance level and peace is restored until the build-up starts again. Examination of such animals reveals hormonal changes that account for some of these actions.

Perhaps it can happen to us—or has it already begun with the rising crime rate, the alienation of so many from society, the increasing incidence of mental illness and consumption of tranquillizers, antidepressants and so forth? We have no way of knowing because, unlike lower animals, we alter our environment in physical and social ways that may make our "space limit" smaller. Slum dwellers come closer to natural conditions and it may start with them. One thing is certain: We in the medical sciences should be thinking seriously about it now. Perhaps we should be demanding an end to the damnable cancerous growth of cities and demanding the formation of new living areas suited to our animal needs for *Lebensraum*. Or maybe we should shut up, knowing that people will not listen, and hope that our children will live to that day when the empty ruins of New York and Rome and Tokyo and Calcutta will echo to the slap of bare feet and the awed chattering of "Homo survivens" coming back from the wilderness.

2. Lippe's Loops and Love

Since prehistoric times, control of population in one way or another has been practiced. Unwanted babies were laid out to die at the edge of settlements in ancient Greece. In some East African countries mothers nursed their babies for two years and the husband was not supposed to consort with this wife until the nursing had ended. Coitus interruptus and other ideas were tried. The industrial age brought in the mechanical devices of which, until recently, the condom was most popular.

Nowadays devices inserted into the uterus have returned to favor in the shape of Lippe's loops or similar space-occupying instruments. In many Western countries sterilization of the female is popular, especially shortly after childbirth when it is easier for both doctor and patient because the uterus is still up out of the pelvis.

With typical timidity or arrogance, males until recently have not looked with favor on being sterilized, although the operation is very simple and not disabling. However in 1971 the Association for Voluntary Sterilization reported that almost 100,000 people a year in the United States are requesting the operation and 78 percent of them are men. In India, persuaded by transistor radios plus sheer desperation, thousands of men are submitting to sterilization, but the effect on the birthrate in that can of worms is hardly noticeable. It is too little and too late.

Rhodesia has been a news item for the last ten years or so, with all sorts of so-called liberals condemning the whites for "brutal suppression" of the blacks. I will say only this about the race-supremacy policy. My houseboy in Malawi had worked in Rhodesia just before he came to me. When we left he went back there because, compared to the black republics, he said Rhodesia offered better pay and better living conditions. He was worried not about freedom to vote but about a decent standard of living. He may have gone back at the wrong time.

The growth rate among the 5 million blacks of Rhodesia is 3.6 percent, almost double that of India. This is because of the medical services provided and largely paid for by the 250,000 white taxpayers. They are rapidly running out of money, and no wonder, when each year there are nearly 200,000 new children to feed, clothe and educate. As it is now, there are not enough jobs for the black people to earn money for their families. They are overgrazing and overcropping their tribal lands. Attempts at a birth-control program are denounced by black politicians as "genocide of blacks by whites." It is against their tribal customs, in any event. The result is a stalemate. In 1968 a world authority on population control told a family-planning seminar in Rhodesia, "In India time has run out, but in Rhodesia you have five minutes more." The five minutes are now gone. Short of governmental enforcement of birth control, which would lead at least to evasion and strikes if not to bloody revolt, the medical profession can only trust in God and get ready for the holocaust. It is bound to come in Africa, but Bangla Desh is beating them to it.

James Barlow, the novelist, put it well in his book *One Man in the World* when he said, re Africa, "Improved health services and schooling escalated the birth and survival rates, but brought near-disaster of a vaster population demanding work but not organized for it. Perhaps the problem was, fundamentally, how to develop a society which would calmly grow crops in a proper manner and do so when it was increasingly disappointed and frustrated by it knew not quite what." He also said, "And Africa was by no means as hot and bothered about so-called freedom as was the white man on its behalf. Some of Africa wasn't enjoying the independence acquired.'' That was several years ago. It is worse today.

In New Guinea, outsiders are amazed to learn that there is a population problem. Overly optimistic health officials who favored an increase of population back in the 1960s and boasted about their antimalaria programs are now beginning to shut up as they wake up to the fact that all this empty land cannot be filled with people. Once forests are cleared off steep slopes, the torrential rains wash away the topsoil in a few years. Then only rank grasses such as kunai survive and the land is good for nothing much but cattle. There is a definite limit to living on such an economy, especially with export markets far away. But the natives keep right on having pickaninnies, as they are called.

Last year two of my colleagues went on a trip to an isolated Highlands area and took movies of the experience. They landed at a little airstrip on a ridge and set up a family-planning clinic for a few days. The word had gone out and they were besieged by thousands of tribesmen, some curious but many wanting help. They inserted Lippe's loops into dozens of *meris* (pidgin for women) who had had five or six children and could not support more. When their supply ran out they flew home, passing over mountain trails crowded with thousands more natives who were too late to be aided.

The acuteness of the problem was illustrated by pictures of whole hillsides denuded of trees, with crude terracing holding small fields of kau-kau (sweet potato) and other vegetables. The shortage of good land has become so acute that in the movie we saw one old lady cultivating a little garden on a seventy-degree slope. It was so steep she had a rope tied to herself and around a bush so she would not fall off her farm.

We all know that the sexual instinct will not be restrained even in our modern cities. We know how to prevent conception, but will we do anything about it? During my five years in Kenya I had an intelligent houseboy. As was customary, his wife lived back in the village tending his land and visited him three or four times a year with the children. Each year, after such a visit, she was pregnant.

The second year he came to me and said, "Bwana, I do not know how I can pay school fees for my two oldest totos [children]."

I gave him a raise in pay and said, "Look, I know the old women of the village tell your wife she should have many children for you, but you cannot educate them and nowadays they *must* be educated to live well. Persuade her to go to the Family Planning Clinic. I will arrange it."

"Ndio, Bwana," he agreed.

That was the last I heard about it until the next child arrived. We repeated the tragicomedy until I left Kenya.

"Bwana," he mourned, "what can I do now?"

"I got you another job," I replied. "I gave you a bonus. You must stop having totos."

"Yes, Bwana, I must."

I passed through Kenya and saw him a year later. There was a new baby.

What we, as doctors, can do about this dreadful inertia I do not know. Custom plus sex drive plus sheer carelessness make a triumvirate that has more power than we do. Someday, perhaps, governments will back us up and make sterilization compulsory. It seems to be the only way short of disaster.

3. The Vice That Became a Virtue

The hypocrisy of human beings is nowhere more evident than in the recent controversy over abortion. When I was a boy in New Zealand my family knew a conscientious young doctor who was well regarded in the community. A girl became pregnant and she and her mother begged him to abort her. He did, but there were complications and the vengeful mother reported him to the police. He was convicted and deprived of his medical license. His life was ruined.

Today what was a crime is encouraged. It is the same sort of hypocrisy we are now seeing in politics with the Chinese Communists. For years when I was in Asia we were forbidden to buy Communist Chinese goods. It was wrong to deal with such immoral people. Today our President has eaten at their table and accepted their gifts. Why is it moral now?

To return to abortions, I am opposed to them, not for moral considerations, but because they are a crude method of population control, psychologically if not physically damaging to millions of women. They, like much surgery, are a confession of failure. I do not like to see life destroyed even where necessary. Prevention is infinitely preferable.

Sometimes there is no other way. In India in 1971 life expectancy had risen from 32 to 52 years and the death rate had dropped from 27.4 per 1,000 to 14 per 1,000. Infant mortality had declined in twenty years from 183 to 113 per 1,000 births. Faced with this increase in population, something had to be done and sterilization and contraception were not enough. There are now 4 million induced abortions each year, 80 percent of them in married women.

Prevention in the form of contraceptives we have discussed above. There is a new way that, if used early enough, is almost as ethically satisfying. I refer to the use of prostaglandins, first used in any quantity in Uganda, East Africa. Now, purists may say that from the moment of conception an egg contains a life that must not be destroyed. I might equally say that the unfertilized ovum is a life, at least a half-life, as is the sperm. They are living human cells too and they die by their millions in the normal processes of procreation without anyone caring. Where religionists draw the line is a matter more of belief, since nobody knows when a human life becomes sentient. Until it does, I feel we can destroy it, if we must, for the common good.

Prostaglandins will prevent the fertilized egg from growing in the uterine mucosa. If it has already become attached and is growing, they will cause changes that will bring on a premature delivery. Done early enough—for example, the morning after intercourse—this will take care of the problem with no more risk to the woman than a normal menstruation. It is far too early to state that this procedure—i.e., hormonal abortion—is free of unwanted side effects, but it almost certainly is no worse than natural abortions which occur in millions every year. The prostaglandins present us with a method which, when mass-produced, will be cheap and easy where we are too lazy to use contraception. We should quit all the silly bickering over legality and get on with it. There is one difficulty: In most countries hormone preparations usually are not issued without a prescription, and this could deny them to about 70 percent of the world's population, according to one expert. Somehow we must get around this barrier while protecting people from possible ill-effects.

4. Killer Kar and the Cowboy Complex

The hysteria over the Vietnam war and the dreadful carnage that was going on over there used to make me nauseated when I read that in ten years of fighting, 50,000 Americans had lost their lives. I was not nauseated by battle casualties—after all, 50,000 men lost their lives in a day in the major battles of the First World War and we lost far more men in the Second World War than in Vietnam. What made me sick was Mama wanting her dear boy safe back home and then gaily waving him off in his new car to kill himself or somebody else on the roads at the rate of 50,000 each year—ten times as many as in Vietnam in a year. Five million were lucky each year—they were only injured. Mama wanted to ban Killer War, but it never occurred to her to stop Killer Kar. And yet the car, in its present form, is one of the most dangerous inventions man has known. It is dangerous in itself (although apologists say the horse was worse per miles traveled) and dangerous for its emissions. It is also dangerous because so much of our good earth has been paved for its use or for reasons which it encourages, thus reducing the green space we need to renew the oxygen we use up each day.

Most people, when they stop to think, realize that cars are a dangerous, uneconomical and slower way to travel, compared with the mass transport systems that could be built right now. They have finally become aware of the dangers of exhaust gas, although not until very recently were they told about the perils of leaded gas used in their souped-up monsters. Now too we find that asbestos particles from scraping brakes may be ruining our lungs. Nobody has yet measured the effects on diseased hearts or twanging nerves of the daily mob scene called commuting to work.

The cowboy complex that makes the car a sublimate for the pinto pony is evident in another of America's great loves—the gun. Unlike the car, it does not enter into everyday life except on television, but it does manage to kill almost half as many people each year. The *New Yorker* of April 20, 1968, stated that since 1900 about 750,000 Americans had been killed by privately owned guns. In 1966 such domestic casualties were 3.5 times greater than Americanmilitary casualties in Vietnam.

To call blasting the guts out of a deer or a duck sport is to reveal a lack of empathy which appears to be a human failing. Such sportsmen should try "shooting" lions or leopards on foot with a camera. The matter is medical in two ways. Firstly, we have to treat the casualties resulting from these love affairs with car and gun. As a pathologist I have to satisfy the police by reassembling the remains and certifying how they died, which perhaps accounts for my aversion. Secondly, having alerted the public to the health problems of air pollution, soil pollution and nerve pollution, we have a never ending duty to remind politicians that we do not need those big cars that put out twice as much dirt as the comfortable and much smaller European types. It has to be politicians because nobody else can tackle the powerful automobile manufacturers. The average American has been so thoroughly brainwashed by advertising in the past twenty-five years that he cannot envision a world where nothing bigger than a Volkswagen with a maximum speed of fifty m.p.h. will be allowed outside of a racetrack. As for guns, almost every other country in the world controls them more stringently than we do.

About 100,000 Americans are killed each year in accidents and 50 million more are injured. Eighteen thousand of these deaths are related to the use of household products and 15,000 are industrial accidents. We pay a high price for our affluence!

5. Advice Is for Someone Else

It is an Irishism to say that if there weren't any people, none of us would have problems. Certainly cutting the world population in half would reduce problems to the point where we might have time to solve them.

After listening for years to those who cry that there are not enough doctors and those there are do not do enough for the public, we in medicine are fighting back. The unpalatable truth is that people themselves are largely responsible for the mess we are in. A Forum on National Health was held in Sun Valley in 1971 and the *American Medical News* reported on July 19, "The most striking conclusion of the forum was that a very large number of Americans are over-doctored, over-hospitalized and over-drugged." I have to agree, especially after seeing how the rest of the world, both developed and not developed, gets on.

In the April 12, 1971, issue of the *Journal of the American Medical Association* it was reported that "nonsickness" among patients visiting doctors in Massachusetts was about 25 percent as compared with 16 percent found in a 1953 study. There is plenty of sickness too, but most of it is caused or made worse by people themselves. I do not refer here to pollution problems. I refer to smoking, getting fat, not taking exercise, eating a poor diet, drinking too much alcohol and so on. Those who get sick from doing these things clutter up our clinics. Accidents are another matter, but it is said 30,000 of the 50,000 deaths due to car accidents each year are associated with drinking. Psychosomatic disease, which I said previously was the commonest cause of sickness in women and high on the list in men is probably greatly aggravated by, if not actually due to, our life habits.

In 1971 John S. Millis, PhD., in the *New England Journal of Medicine* said in part, "Far too many people regard health as being 'doctored.' They therefore hope that with the right to unlimited access to physicians and hospitals, they will all be healthy." Later he said, "We accept the concept that health is a necessity but realize that we, as a society, can guarantee only access to health services. Personal health must remain a personal responsibility . . . we must convince people that the achievement of health demands responsibility and action on the part of each individual."

At about the same time an article in the *Journal of the Indiana State Medical Association* said, "Most of our citizens are interested in preventive medicine and good health if someone else produces its benefits. Very few people are interested in their own welfare enough to work for it." And later, "Suicide by eating too much, suffocation by cigarettes, and homicide by careless auto driving are three diseases that are typical of what the American public thinks of preventive medicine. They don't want any of it and will not use it when it is available." That is pretty tough talk—unpalatable medicine, but necessary.

A side issue here, mentioned before, is the public's aversion to protective immunizations—perhaps not so much aversion as indifference. Not long ago it was decided in the United States to abolish smallpox vaccinations on the grounds that there is now no smallpox in the States and there have been a very few deaths from the vaccines. While this is true, it tends to give us a false sense of security, a security that could suddenly vanish in these days of rapid and frequent travel. In April 1972, after this ruling was made, an epidemic of smallpox broke out in Yugoslavia which had been free of it for years. The disease was brought back by a Muslim who had been on a pilgrimage to Mecca. Twenty-nine employees of the hospital where he was sent got the disease before the danger was realized, and the infection was spread to Germany by a migrant worker. Four people have died at the time I write this.

It is my feeling that the medical profession is pandering to public apathy when allowing inoculations and vaccinations to be voluntary. In Canada during the Second World War I saw scores of victims of infectious disease, such as diphtheria, among soldiers who had not had preventive inoculations or had allowed them to lapse. The epidemics arose and spread with frightening rapidity as troops moved from one base to another. They could arise again today and travel as fast as a jet around the world.

6. Oh, Happy Breed!

One of the tenets of the modern materialistic society is that happiness is a commodity and can be bought. If only we provide everybody with what he wants, then we should all be at least content. It is not necessarily so.

My wife tells me of visiting a friend, the daughter of a millionaire, when they were both young girls. My wife was a minister's daughter, not too well off in the Depression. She was excited about the possibility of getting something she really wanted for Christmas. When she talked about it the rich girl said, "How lucky you are! Christmas doesn't excite me at all. I have everything I can ask for."

Today the people of Sweden are getting to that stage. They are cushioned by their socialist state against want. They have medical care, old-age pensions, good working hours and so on—all the things a socialist utopia should provide. And what is the result?

Sweden has one of the highest suicide rates in the world. The number of inpatients in mental institutions rose from 73,000 in 1969 to 83,000 in 1970. In 1972 a report commissioned by the national social-welfare authorities and written by Dr. Hans Lohmann, a psychiatrist, was published. It pointed to the vicious cycle in which a high rate of economic growth is necessary to pay the cost of looking after those who cannot keep up, but as their number steadily increases, a higher growth rate is needed, and the end is a spiral up into futility. The report paints a gloomy picture of a merciless, unfriendly society and concludes that a country's welfare can no longer be measured simply by its standard of life and that the Swedes are increasingly sacrificing their mental health for improvements in their material environment. Put simply, by the time they are millionaires they will all be mad.

The same situation holds throughout the Western world, the report claims, and I certainly agree. The suicide rate in Los Angeles for ages 20 to 29 was 12.2 per 100,000 in 1960. In 1969 it had risen to 28.4 per 100,000. Drugs were not the cause. Fears of parental pressure and a feeling of loneliness were major factors. The medical profession should be taking the lead in turning away from our obsession with things. Many youngsters are already doing so. Christ told us to do it 2,000 years ago, but we have not listened.

7. Home, Sweet Nursing Home

Almost everybody takes care of kids, but almost nobody wants to take care of old people. In 1971 the Senate Special Committee on Aging reported that one out of every four Americans sixty-five or older was living on a poverty-level income. There were 4.8 million of them living in poverty in 1969, an increase of almost 200,000 since the previous year. A recent hospital survey in New York revealed that out of 18,102 hospital beds, 1,513 were occupied by "holdovers." These were mostly elderly people who had no place to go for the convalescent care they needed. At $100 per day, the average cost of a hospital bed in New York City, it was costing $55 million a year to keep these people in hospitals.

In an article on "Effective Management of Health" in the *British Medical Journal* of May 29, 1971 it was stated that "At present 40 percent of all bed days in hospital are used by pensioners and 38 percent of all hospital costs. By the year 2000 the first figure could be 80 percent." It has also been reported that there is severe overcrowding, understaffing and inadequate toilet facilities in British hospitals where geriatric, chronic sick and mental cases are treated.

During the 1960s in the United States the population in the age-group 5 to 24 rose by 28 percent. In the age group 65 and over it rose 21 percent, but in the group 25 to 44 it expanded by less than 3 percent. This means that, in proportion, fewer people are now taking care of an increasing number of those too young to work and those too old to be of much use. The recent drop in the American birthrate, if sustained, will relieve the taxpayer of some of the burden of the young but not, for a long time, of the old.

Today in Ameriia there are more than 20 million people sixty-five or older and there will be about 25 million in 1980. Life expectancy, which was 47 in my father's day, is now 86.2, according to Vincent Wallen, Ph.D., Chief of the Psychology Service of the Veterans Administration Hospital in Hampton, Virginia. His figure seems about ten years too high to mc and I havc no way of checking it. Even so, the difference is enormous. It is not that people who reach the age of forty-five live longer than they did in 1900, but that more people survive past the first half-century than ever before. In an article in *Military Medicine*, November 1970, Dr. Wallen stated, "The present way of dealing with the aged seems to be making sure there aren't too many of them around. Our society in general tends to isolate them, to restrict their activities, and to encourage their leaving the labor market. The family tends to put the aged member in his place, usually a nursing home or a rest home. Such a placement invariably cuts off almost completely the emotional, social and physical ties that have been previously established, nurtured, and developed over many years.

Thus from sixty-five to a wished-for death at eighty-five plus (or seventy-five plus?) we are condemning our old people to a sort of prison, not quite as bad as solitary confinement, but cutting them off from activity, from involvement with the world as they know it. This, in a more severe form, is essentially what the Communists did to American prisoners in the Korean War when they wanted to break them down. Young men cracked under the strain. How can we expect the old ones to do better? We are, in fact, creating sick people who, in Dr. Wallen's words, "sit . . . staring off into space in modern air-conditioned rooms, mumbling to themselves, ignoring everything going on around them, expecting and receiving total care, and not having any responsibilities other than breathing, swallowing, and defecating. In such a setting, injury rates, intercurrent illnesses, and problem behaviors run high.'' As I said earlier, man is an animal, and if you want to see what we are doing to the old people, go to any badly run zoo and watch the bears and wolves and cats pace back and forth in their little prisons. If you still need convincing, listen to Dr. Frederick C. Swartz, Chairman of the American Medical Association's Committee on Aging. He said in 1972, ''Compulsory retirement based on age without regard for the individual's desire and ability to continue work can be a prime factor in health deterioration of the retiree.'' He added that the suicide rate in males over sixty is the highest of any age group.

Contrast this with what I saw back in 1957 when I arrived in Taiwan with the U.S. Army. We were given a small house on the outskirts of Taipei where there were rice paddies all about. Near our house was a little village and beyond our back fence was a family compound where we could see and hear the life of a typical Chinese farmer group family. There were the patriarchal grandfather and his wife, whose feet had been bound for a while in her girlhood so that she walked awkwardly, flat-footed and toes turned out. There were middle-aged sons and their families, young newlyweds and, all over the place from early morning to late at night, big kids, little kids, toddlers and babies, running, playing, fighting, crying or squalling for the breast.

When the sun shone, grandmother waddled about outside, supervising and scolding. Grandfather sat smoking his long bamboo pipe, a crawler at his feet and little ones playing around him, coming to him for help, for comfort, for companionship. Everybody belonged, everybody had a place. It was not idyllic, of course. There were intrigues and jealousies, problems of all kinds, but all the family members were busy, all were involved, and the old people were *alive*.

It is not possible to return to a life as simple as we have abandoned, but it has advantages. For instance, villagers in Bulgaria, Soviet Georgia and Hunza in India often live to great ages. A report in August 1971 from a village in Ecuador stated that it happens in the New World as well. Of 800 people in the village, 38 were over 75. Several were over 100. One old man was 121 years old and a woman 109. Both ages were confirmed from church records.

These people lived on beans, unpolished rice and vegetables and fruit. They had meat once or twice a week. They remained physically active in the fields or at their trades. In other words, they remained part of the community and were not put aside to wither away.

Except for a few old-fashioned villages in the rural areas, we of the marvelous materialistic society havc lost all this. And we are paying dearly for it. Expensive nursing homes, group therapy with clinical psychologists and so forth all help to keep the patients going, but they tend to remain patients or to relapse. It is true that a senile parent, partly crippled by a stroke, can be a terrible burden on a family if at home. Such people need to be in hospitals or homes, or, if we ever get to it, disposed of by an euthanasia committee. They are not the majority. The failure of doctors, families and communities to accept responsibility for making the last part of life as comfortable and happy as possible makes a mockery of our moral preaching. We forget that our turn will come and we are making our own hell.

14

Ecology —The New Medicine

1. We Are All Involved in Everything

If writing this book has brought me to any conclusion, it is this: Medicine is misdirected because for too long it has emphasized cure rather than prevention. All through medical or nursing school or any other type of paramedical training we hear what to do about diseases, once people catch them. We do have some teaching on prevention, but it is of lesser importance in the minds of all but those who take up preventive medicine as a specialty. Even they, until very recently, have had a skewed vision of what needs to be done. Part of this is because they have been told by politicians and others, "Medicine is too important to be left to the doctors," whereupon the politician and special pleaders get millions for their pet projects. Doctors do the same, with malariologists competing with infectious-disease experts and cancer researchers for funds and all shouldering aside the newcomer, the family-planning expert.

What none of these people realized is that we are living in an incredibly complex environment where one action may trigger off a totally unexpected result, not obvious until we look at it from another viewpoint. For example, an asbestos worker has seven to ten times more chance of getting cancer of the lungs than another worker, but if he smokes, the risk is eighty to ninety times greater. The Aswan Dam fiasco is another example of unexpected results and it should teach us not to make plans in isolation from all the facts. Whether we like it or not, we are all involved and interlinked into one great ecosystem. When we understand better how the system works, we should be able to prevent much of the disease that troubles us today.

In a special article in *Modern Medicine* (Australian edition, February 21, 1972) Dr. John J. Hanlon, Assistant Surgeon General, Public Health Service of the United States, noted that Hippocrates, and others later, recognized clearly the intimacy of the man-environment relationship. He went on to say, "However, when scientific and technological medicine began its ascendancy, diseases came to be regarded increasingly as phenomena quite unto themselves, wholly intrinsic or internal with regard to cause, consequence or cure." Later he said, "The essential fallacy of this approach was that it overlooked the fact that man, his environment, and all the other things in it were really all inter-dependent parts of the same thing—the ecosystem."

2. The Physical Aspects

When I talked about the diseases of civilization I said we already knew how to prevent them, although I admitted I could not explain exactly why some of them occurred. All that is necessary is a return to a more basic way of life, combined with a clean environment and a smaller population—in other words, get back to where physical evolution had brought us before our social evolution literally gummed up the works.

Now, this is a very unpopular idea. Few people want to give up their steaks, butter, ice cream, cookies, drinks, smokes and cars. They don't want to pay the price for clean air, clean water, clean land. They will wait for the new pill to lower blood pressure and serum cholesterol, the pill that will dissolve the fatty plaques in their arteries, the substitute cigarette and coffee that will not constrict their arteries, the harmless drink that tastes and acts like Scotch. And while there is "Growthandprogress," a multiple word that should be declared obscene, they will continue to fight like warring ants for supremacy in the material world, stressing beyond endurance their rusty pipes and short-circuiting nervous system. It is a pity this is so, but because it is, 75 percent of all Americans —in fact, 75 percent of all peoples called "developed"—will die before their time. There is no wonder drug for all this. We need environmental control of our physical world.

That is where medicine should have its future. But can we enforce such discipline? I can't get my own wife to give up smoking, so I do not have much hope. At least I keep my family out of cities and in the clean air of primitive countries. Perhaps the American businessman can be forced to clean up his mess. Perhaps the American taxpayer will pay for his part of it. Perhaps.

In considering the great diseases that plague the undeveloped world—malaria, schistosomiasis, TB and so on—we must rethink our medical attack on ecological lines and we must be hard-hearted about it. I see no use eliminating malaria to replace it with malnutrition due to overpopulation. Equally, I see no use in eliminating malnutrition (as in providing more rice fields at Aswan) only to cripple people with schistosomiasis or malaria. I see no use in cutting down the death rate in newborn babies, as one WHO doctor proudly reported from Laos, only to have war injuries, cholera and starvation carry them off a year or so later. Until we can control populations we should not control the diseases that are natural curbs. If we do, we are making certain of that dreadful day when ten or a hundred times as many people perish in wars and famines brought on by population pressure. We are then, in the Biblical phrase, visiting our sins upon our children. It is happening today in Bangla Desh.

To turn to research, I often feel—and I am in good company—that it is time for a partial moratorium. With what we have already discovered, properly used, we can eliminate most of the world's medical problems. But we do not do it. It is like our defense program. We already can blow any enemy to hell, and ourselves with him, but we go on spending billions to refine further our overkill program.

And why not have a moratorium? What is this *truth that must be sought*? Why must it be? Who demands it, outside of the directly interested scientist? To say that we will regress if we do not progress is a bit of semireligious cant that is dragged out by researchers whenever the subject comes up. To quash that argument, all we have to do is to look at nature. Living things grow to maturity and then, for a long time relative to the time it took to reach maturity, they remain in balance. After that they decay. We are at the stage where if we do not achieve a balance, if we keep on growing, we are no longer a normal ecosystem but a cancerous one that will destroy itself by its own growth. So I say let us pause awhile to reflect, and then if we think we need more research, more growth, we can have it in strictly controlled doses.

3. The Mental Aspects

In considering the mental aspects of the New Medicine, I start with education. As I said above, our emphasis in medicine until now has been on cure rather than prevention. The same is true in our medical schools, and it must end. Let us try to look at it dispassionately.

If we spent as much money on safety measures as we spend on treating the millions of accidents each year, we could probably cut out most of the injuries and cut back the load on our casualty clinics. A simple medical treatment or, better still, a vaccine for viruses in cancer would eliminate the need for thousands of hospital beds and many of our staff. Then we would be free to turn our attention to the mental diseases which are becoming our greatest problem.

Ah ha, you say, but you said cut down on research! So I did, on uncontrolled repetitive research in the physical aspects of medicine, churning out millions of useless statistics and medical articles. We need to be ruthless with our thinking and our priorities in research. Prevention of disease in all its aspects must have a high priority, and our education must be biased along those lines.

Another place where education is sorely needed is in the utilization of medical services. We need to alter the thinking of doctors and, even more, the thinking of people. Even the poorest countries, where free medical care is a sop to the people, waste their medical personnel on frivolous complaints. Americans are among the worst wasters of medical talent in the world, and it is time they were made to realize it. Socialization of medical services is not the answer, either to the cost of medical care to the people or to the so-called doctor shortage. If anything, it is often more wasteful of money and manpower. What is needed is discipline. Medical care is a limited resource and it must be carefully rationed and used. We doctors can help, but this is mainly a people problem—a problem of mental attitudes.

Looking into the future, I foresee that the New Medicine will have one role above all others: the adjustment of man's mentality to bring it into balance with nature. I cannot say how many of the psychiatric illnesses that worry us today are the result of our getting out of step with nature, but I suspect most of them. We seem to be getting beyond our mental and emotional capacity to handle the problems created by our social evolution. Perhaps if we doctors study mental disease from the ecological viewpoint and if we can get people to follow our recommendations, we will be able to empty mental hospitals of most of the load by remaking the world into one that overstressed minds can cope with.

4. The Moral Aspects

The medical moral problem of greatest immediacy today is abortion. It is said that necessity is the mother of invention. It is also the mother of morals and led, in the past, to the prohibition of eating pork or beef, to laws against incest and to other taboos. Sometimes it works the other way, allowing certain acts rather than prohibiting them. Thus we might think of polygamy and polyandry as moral or immoral depending on our cultural heritage, which has been conditioned by the necessities of the past. So it is with abortion.

To me, killing a pre-sentient fetus to control population is a much more moral act than killing soldiers to preserve one's territory or so-called national integrity. Yet until recently governments balked at the former and encouraged the latter. Why make such a fuss over abortion when we know the misery that will be prevented by allowing it? If we must apportion guilt, let it be to a society that is too short-sighted to take more acceptable contraceptive measures, and to those persistent offenders too lazy or ignorant or careless to use easily available personal measures of prevention. I do not mean to use measures such as shame or prosecution. I mean such measures as doing away with tax exemptions and baby bonuses for children. In the future we may have to issue licenses to have children and order compulsory sterilization for those who will not comply with directives to limit the number. Some will consider this an infringement of individual liberties and therefore immoral, but, in the ecological view of morals, those who overcrowd the world are the real sinners against mankind.

There are other ecological moral problems for the future. Will it be right, for instance, to continue to treat patients and use overworked facilities in cases where the disease is brought about by their own acts? Let us consider the heavy smoker cluttering up a bed as a chronic emphysema patient. Does he have the right to our services? After the first coronary attack will the heart-disease sufferer get into the Intensive Care Unit for the second attack if he has failed to follow our recommendations on diet, medication and so on? Why should he not stay home and take his chances while we use the facilities for a first offender? If the unit were full of such people, how would we feel if a gravely ill child could not be accommodated? It may yet come to that.

I realize that the above sounds as if I were talking about criminals by calling coronary patients first offenders. I am assuming here that the medical profession and health departments will have educated people to the dangers of their way of life as they are now doing about smoking. It sounds callous, I know, but I must insist that those who continue smoking today are, if they become ill from its effects, guilty of a self-inflicted wound and so are as guilty as any other attempted suicide. If we consider suicidal people as psychiatric problems and drop the prosecution that now exists in law, then I would agree to call such lung- and heart-disease sufferers psychiatric cases too. However, I still insist they should not have priority for treatment when the day comes that we no longer can afford to keep building, equipping and staffing our superhospitals.

That day will assuredly come if people keep on demanding more and more treatment but do not want to tax themselves enough to pay for it. There is another moral problem here, especially under socialism. Why should the taxpayer carry the load not only for his own diseases but also for the equally self-inflicted diseases of the poorer people who do not pay taxes? Does not the poor man have to pay something for his negligence? This is especially the problem in undeveloped countries and one which will eventually break down their medical services when the tax base cannot support the load. I have always said that families of the poor sick person can pay something. If not money, they can pay in labor for the government, donate blood and so on; but they must pay in some way for their right to live.

5. The World Is Our Patient

We must all pay for the right to live on our planet. It is not only a moral obligation, it is now an ecological necessity if we are to survive. We have been obsessed for too long with our interpersonal relationships in medicine, with our curing of individual diseases, with our mechanical miracles and our esoteric research. We have ignored the great ecological problems that threaten to overwhelm us. We have poisoned ourselves with our "Growth-and progress" excesses and we have failed to notice what has happened to our minds in the process of becoming "civilized."

This we have done as people. Those concerned with medicine in the broad sense, doctors, nurses, clergy, politicians and others, have failed to give the right lead on the path to a better life. They have taken us up blind alleys and through dangerous short cuts. We are now well on the way to disaster if we do not stop and think. Only thus will we save our patient, the world, and, as part of the world, ourselves.

Max Nicholson in his book *The Environmental Revolution: A Guide for the New Masters of the Earth* said, "It is now a commonplace that we are currently experiencing another of these decisive shifts of initiative and power, in which the technocrat is progressively, although gropingly and hesitantly, stepping into the shoes of earlier ruling types. This replacement is essential and indeed badly overdue. *Even in relation to environmental management alone the capability of a classically educated group of administrators and politicians for handling the new forces and tools here outlined is little better than that of a band of apes faced with the task of devising an agricultural system.*" [Italics mine.]

We in the medical field are technocrats. If Max Nicholson is right, and I believe he is, we should be demanding change —demanding a new group of officers on space-ship Earth who can change its course and avert disaster.

Will we do it in time?

INDEX